MIKE BARREL

Eat to Live vs. Live to Eat:

Reclaim Your Health and Transform Your Relationship with Food

First edition

This book was professionally typeset on Reedsy.
Find out more at reedsy.com

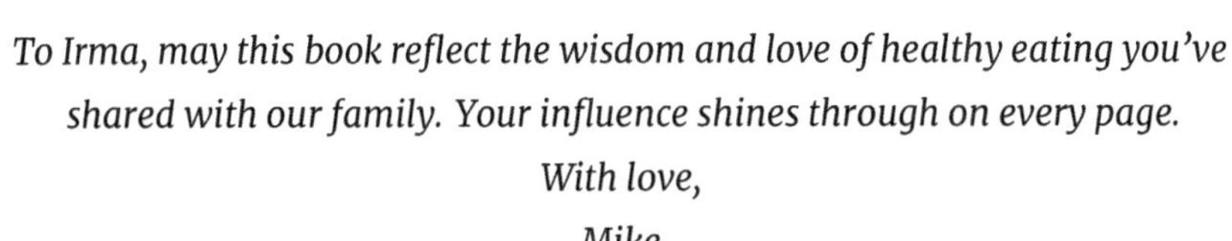

To Irma, may this book reflect the wisdom and love of healthy eating you've shared with our family. Your influence shines through on every page.
With love,
Mike

Contents

Introduction   1

The Crossroads of Convenience and Consequence   1

Chapter 1: Understanding the Enemies – Unveiling the Hidden...   4

Section 1: Processed Foods – Beyond Simple Preparation   6

Section 2: Toxic Ingredients – Unmasking the Dangers in Your Food   9

Section 3: The Industry and Misleading Labels – Don't Be Deceived   13

Chapter 2: The Detox Plan – Resetting Your Body for Optimal...   16

Section 1: The Elimination Phase – A Path to Personalized Nutrition   19

Section 2: Hydration – The Essential Flow for Detoxification   22

Section 3: Natural Detox Support – Harnessing the Power of Nature   25

Chapter 3: The Maintenance Plan – Nourishing Your Body for...   28

Section 1: Embracing Whole Foods – Building Blocks for Optimal Health   31

Section 2: Meal Planning and Practicality – Integrating Healthy Eating into Your Lifestyle   34

Section 3: Portion Control & Mindful Eating – Reconnecting with Your Body's Wisdom   37

Chapter 4: Food for Life – Finding Freedom and Lasting...   40

Section 1: Emotional Eating and Mindful Solutions
– Breaking the Cycle   42

Section 2: Building Sustainable Habits – Embracing
the Journey   45

Section 3: Social Navigation – Maintaining Your
Healthy Path   48

Chapter 5: Exercise – Adding Movement to Your Routine   51

Section 1: The Benefits of Exercise – Your Prescription for a Healthier, Happier Life   54

Section 2: Designing Your Fitness Plan – Discover
the Joy of Movement   57

Section 3: Getting Started – Your Journey to a More
Active Life   60

Conclusion   63

Appendix A: Recipes   66

Breakfast   67

Lunch   73

Dinner   80

Snacks   86

Recipes Designed with Adaptability in Mind   90

Appendix B:Food Swaps   95

Appendix C: Glossary of Nutritional Terms   100

Appendix D: Recommended Resources   103

About the Author   106

Introduction

The Crossroads of Convenience and Consequence

Food in Modern Society

The modern era has brought with it a relentless pursuit of convenience. Time has become a precious commodity, leading us to seek out shortcuts for nearly every aspect of our lives, including food. The allure of ready-made meals, packaged snacks, and drive-thru windows promises instant gratification. Sadly, this convenience comes at a heavy price – the decline of natural, whole-food eating. Once-treasured traditions of home-cooked meals shared around tables have been replaced by hastily consumed, nutrient-poor options, often eaten in isolation.

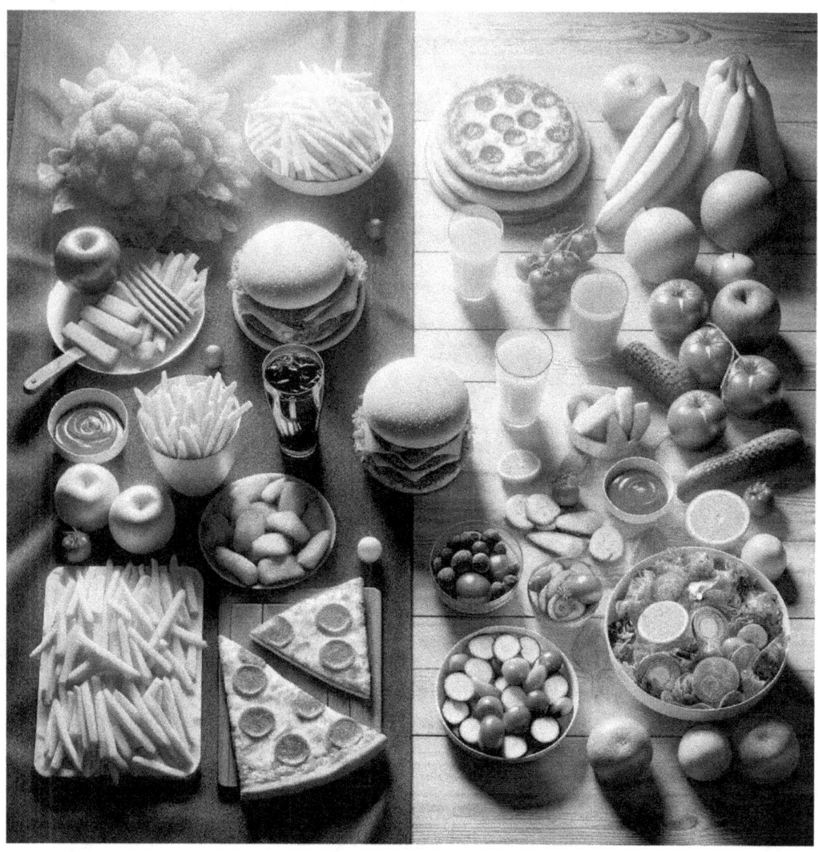

Simultaneously, we're witnessing a startling explosion of chronic diseases. The connection between diet and disease is undeniable. As processed foods loaded with harmful ingredients flood our supermarkets, our bodies struggle to cope. Chronic inflammation, a silent but destructive process, lurks at the root of many modern health problems. Additionally, the stripping away of vital nutrients in processed foods leaves our bodies lacking the essential building blocks for optimal health.

"Live to Eat" vs. "Eat to Live"

Modern society has cultivated an unhealthy obsession with food as a source of pleasure. Advertisements bombard us with tantalizing images and engineered flavors designed to trigger cravings and override our natural hunger signals. Food becomes a means of entertainment, comfort, and social status, rather than simply a source of nourishment. The mantra of "Live to Eat" perpetuates the notion that food's primary purpose is to provide sensory pleasure, often at the expense of our health.

In stark contrast, "Eat to Live" presents a profoundly different perspective. This principle recognizes that food is, first and foremost, fuel for our bodies. It's about choosing whole, unprocessed foods that deliver the vitamins, minerals, and antioxidants necessary for optimal health, longevity, and disease prevention. While taste and enjoyment are still important factors, they take a back seat to the nutritional value of our choices.

This book serves as a guide to navigating this shifting landscape. You'll learn to discern between the empty promises of the processed food world and the true power of whole-food nourishment. The "Eat to Live" way isn't about deprivation, but empowerment. It's about discovering the profound satisfaction that comes from fueling your body with what it needs to thrive. Join the transformation toward a healthier, more vibrant you.

Chapter 1: Understanding the Enemies – Unveiling the Hidden Dangers of Modern Food

In the battle for your health, knowledge is your most potent weapon. This chapter arms you with the critical understanding needed to identify the insidious enemies lurking within our food supply. We'll dissect the deceptive world of processed foods, expose the dangers of toxic ingredients, and empower you to see through the misleading tactics of the food industry.

First, let's clarify what we mean by "processed" and "ultra-processed" foods. These aren't simply foods that have undergone some preparation. The real culprits are foods stripped of their natural goodness, and then laden with artificial ingredients, refined sugars, unhealthy fats, and a host of additives. You'll learn to recognize them in their many disguises: ready-to-eat meals, sugary cereals, salty snacks, refined grains, and countless other seemingly harmless items crowding supermarket shelves.

Understanding the mechanisms of harm is crucial. These foods wreak havoc on your body, triggering blood sugar spikes and crashes that lead to cravings, weight gain, and eventually, chronic diseases like diabetes.

They ravage your gut microbiome – the foundation of our immune system – leaving you vulnerable to digestive problems, inflammation, and even mood disorders. As if this wasn't enough, these foods are nutritionally bankrupt, offering little more than empty calories that displace the vitamins and minerals your body craves.

We'll also shine a spotlight on toxic ingredients commonly used to improve taste, texture, and shelf life. From artificial sweeteners with questionable health consequences to trans fats that raise your risk of heart disease, you'll gain the knowledge to spot these red flags. High fructose corn syrup, a ubiquitous sweetener linked to metabolic dysfunction, will be thoroughly examined. And, we won't forget the dangers of added sugars, silent drivers of inflammation, and a major contributor to countless health problems. Finally, we'll discuss the murky world of food dyes and additives, exploring potential links to cancer and gut health disturbances.

The food industry is skilled in the art of deception. They use clever marketing ploys and "health halos" to make unhealthy products appear virtuous. You'll master deciphering those misleading labels and learn to read ingredient lists with a detective's eye. Don't be fooled by macronutrient counts (protein, fat, carbs) alone – true nutrition goes much deeper.

By the end of this chapter, you'll emerge with a newfound clarity. No longer will you be a passive victim of cleverly marketed products. Instead, you'll be an empowered, informed consumer, ready to make food choices that protect and nourish your health for the long term.

Section 1: Processed Foods – Beyond Simple Preparation

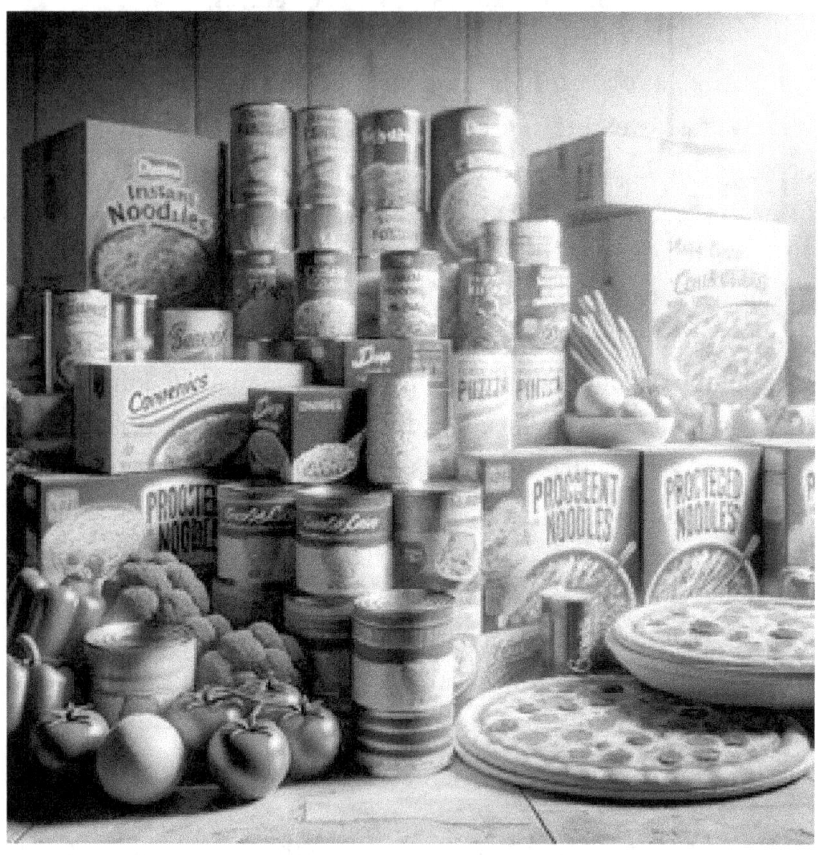

When we discuss "processed foods," we're not merely referring to foods that have undergone some form of preparation. Washing an apple or cutting vegetables for a salad are examples of beneficial processing. The danger lies in the transformation of whole foods into products that bear little resemblance to their original state. Let's dive into the key terms:

- **Processed Foods:** These have been altered from their natural state through processes like canning, freezing, milling, or drying. While some minimally processed foods can be healthy choices (think frozen vegetables or canned beans), many go much further. They include added sugars, refined oils, artificial flavors, colors, and preservatives.
- **Ultra-Processed Foods:** This category represents the worst offenders. They're often concoctions of industrial ingredients, engineered for maximum convenience and shelf-life, not health. These products are typically high in calories, sodium, unhealthy fats, and refined carbohydrates, yet devoid of real nutrition.

Categories and Examples: Spotting the Culprits

- **Ready-to-Eat Meals:** Frozen pizzas, microwavable dinners, and canned pasta laden with sodium and preservatives fall into this category.
- **Snack Foods:** Think chips, crackers, cookies, pastries, and candy bars. These offer little more than empty calories, sugary bursts, and unhealthy fats.
- **Refined Grains:** White bread, white rice, and most breakfast cereals are stripped of their fiber and essential nutrients, with added sugars frequently tossed in.
- **Sugary Drinks:** Sodas, sweetened teas, sports drinks, and fruit-flavored beverages deliver massive doses of sugar with no nutritional value.

Mechanisms of Harm: The Assault on Your Body

1. **Blood Sugar Dysregulation:** Ultra-processed foods often contain refined carbohydrates and added sugars that cause rapid spikes in blood sugar levels, followed by a crash. This roller coaster disrupts metabolic health, leading to increased hunger, cravings, and weight gain. Over time, chronic blood sugar imbalances significantly raise your risk for type 2 diabetes, heart disease, and metabolic disorders.
2. **Gut Microbiome Damage:** Your gut is home to trillions of microorganisms that play vital roles in digestion, immunity, and overall health. Ultra-processed foods, with their lack of fiber, additives, and emulsifiers, disrupt the delicate balance of your gut bacteria. This imbalance is linked to a multitude of health problems, including:

- Digestive issues: bloating, constipation, diarrhea
- Weakened immune system
- Increased inflammation
- Mood disturbances (due to the gut-brain connection)

1. **Nutrient Deficiencies:** As ultra-processed foods displace whole foods in your diet, your body is deprived of essential vitamins, minerals, and antioxidants. These deficiencies can manifest in various ways:

- Fatigue and weakness
- Poor immune function
- Impaired mental clarity
- Increased risk for disease development

Key Takeaway: Ultra-processed foods are designed to stimulate taste buds, not nourish your body. They offer short-term satisfaction at the expense of long-term health. By understanding the true nature of these foods and how they sabotage your well-being, you'll be empowered to make choices that fuel your health instead of fueling disease.

Section 2: Toxic Ingredients – Unmasking the Dangers in Your Food

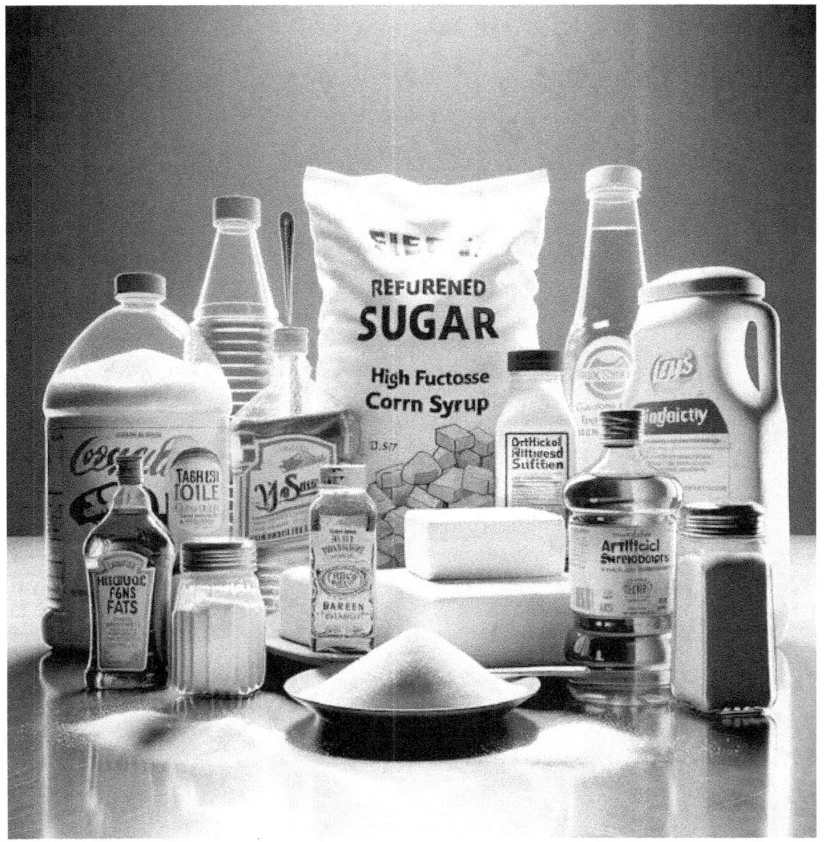

Picture this: you decide to treat yourself to a "sugar-free" dessert, assuming it's a healthier choice. However, a deep dive into the ingredients reveals a list of artificial sweeteners, additives, and other processed components. This seemingly innocent swap might be sabotaging your health goals more than you realize. Let's demystify the most common toxic ingredients you must learn to spot:

Artificial Sweeteners (aspartame, sucralose, etc.): The Bitter Truth

- The Promise: Intense sweetness with zero calories, a tempting proposition for weight control and blood sugar management.
- The Reality: Artificial sweeteners disrupt our bodies in unexpected ways:
- **Gut Bacteria Imbalance:** Research suggests they negatively impact the balance of beneficial bacteria in our digestive system, potentially contributing to metabolic issues and weakened immunity.
- **Increased Food Cravings:** Confusing your brain's natural hunger and satiety signals, artificial sweeteners might lead to overeating and a constant desire for something sweet.
- **Potential Blood Sugar Spikes:** Though marketed as blood-sugar friendly, there's evidence some artificial sweeteners might still trigger an insulin response, negating their intended benefit.
- **Long-term Safety Concerns:** Some studies raise questions about potential links to cancer risk, though we need more definitive human research.

Trans Fats (hydrogenated oils): Heart Attack on a Plate

- The Purpose: Created to solidify oils and extend shelf life, they were once ubiquitous in snacks, baked goods, and fried foods.
- The Health Fallout: Trans fats are the undisputed villains of the

nutrition world. They dramatically raise LDL ("bad") cholesterol and lower HDL ("good") cholesterol, significantly increasing your risk of heart disease, stroke, and type 2 diabetes.

- Important Note: Due to FDA regulations, most trans fats have been banned from processed foods. However, always scan the ingredient lists, as they might linger in older products or those made in countries with less stringent regulations.

High Fructose Corn Syrup (HFCS): A Sweet Path to Disease

- The Prevalence: HFCS is a cheap, highly processed sweetener that has infiltrated our food supply, showing up in everything from sodas and candy to bread and condiments.
- The Damage: Our bodies metabolize HFCS differently than regular sugar. It burdens the liver heavily, leading to:
- **Fat Accumulation:** HFCS promotes the storage of fat, particularly in the liver, contributing to fatty liver disease and belly fat.
- **Insulin Resistance:** It disrupts how our bodies use insulin, the hormone regulating blood sugar. This leads to a higher risk of type 2 diabetes and metabolic syndrome.
- **Inflammation:** HFCS triggers chronic inflammation, the foundation of many modern health problems.

Added Sugars: Fueling the Flames of Inflammation

- The Hidden Invasion: Added sugars sneak into countless foods— yogurts, salad dressings, sauces, cereals, "healthy" snack bars, and more.
- The Health Consequences: Constant excessive sugar intake drives chronic, low-grade inflammation throughout the body. Over time, inflammation contributes to:

- Heart Disease
- Type 2 Diabetes
- Certain types of Cancer
- Autoimmune Conditions
- Obesity
- Cognitive Decline

Food Dyes and Additives: A Murky Cloud of Uncertainty

- The Purpose: To enhance color, flavor, and texture, preserve freshness, and mask inferior ingredients.
- The Concerns: While many additives are deemed "generally recognized as safe" (GRAS), some are cause for concern:
- Food Dyes: Some artificial colors may have links to hyperactivity and attention problems in children.
- Certain Preservatives: Some may be possible carcinogens and could be linked to digestive issues.
- Gut Health Impact: Many additives could disrupt the balance of our gut microbiome, with potential consequences on overall health.
- The Bottom Line: More research is needed, but opting for foods with short, simple ingredient lists is always a healthier choice.

Key Takeaway: Be a conscious consumer! Educate yourself on these toxic ingredients to make informed choices that support your health, not hinder it.

Section 3: The Industry and Misleading Labels – Don't Be Deceived

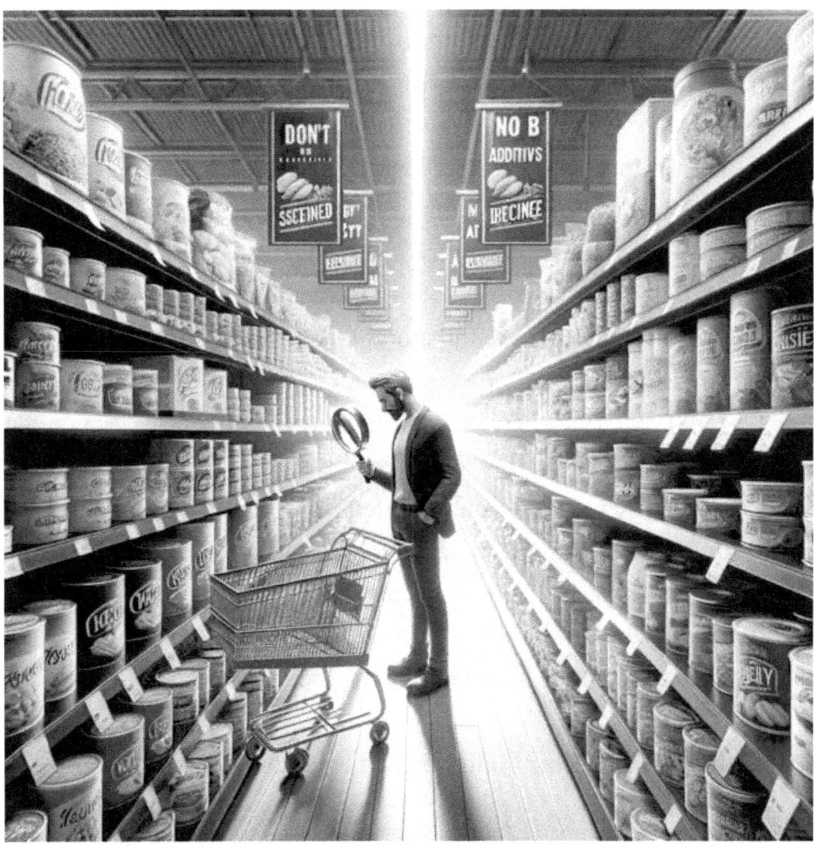

The processed food industry has mastered the art of manipulation, using clever buzzwords, misleading packaging, and targeted marketing to give unhealthy products a deceptive aura of health. It's crucial to become a savvy consumer who sees through these tactics, so you can make empowered food choices aligned with your health goals.

Deciphering "Health Halos"

- The Strategy: Terms like "low-fat," "sugar-free," "gluten-free," "natural," or "organic" create an illusion of health and often distract from the overall nutritional profile.
- The Reality: Here's how these terms can mislead:
- **Low-Fat:** Often, fat is replaced with added sugar, refined carbs, and excess salt, leaving the product nutritionally void.
- **Sugar-Free:** Doesn't mean calorie-free. These products often rely on artificial sweeteners, with their own potential health drawbacks, and might still contain high amounts of unhealthy fats or refined carbohydrates.
- **Gluten-Free:** While necessary for those with Celiac disease or gluten intolerance, this label doesn't mean healthy. Gluten-free snacks can be highly processed and deficient in vital nutrients.
- **Natural:** Sadly, this term is loosely regulated. Highly processed foods can sometimes still carry this label.
- **Organic:** While organic foods generally have fewer pesticide residues, "organic" junk food is still junk food.

Marketing Tactics: Don't Judge a Food by its Packaging

- Appealing Images: Pictures of wholesome ingredients like fresh fruits and vegetables on a highly processed product can create a false sense of health.
- Buzzwords and Slogans: Catchy phrases like "wholesome" or "made with real fruit" are designed to trigger positive associations, while obscuring the reality of the product.

Understanding Ingredient Lists and Nutrition Labels: Your Defense Against Deception

- Reading Beyond Macros: Calories, protein, fat, and carbs are important but don't tell the whole story. Here's where your focus should be:
- **Ingredient List:** Ingredients are listed in order by weight. Are the first few ingredients whole foods or a litany of processed components and additives? The fewer items on the list and the more recognizable they are, the better.
- **Added Sugars:** Check under the "Carbohydrates" section on the nutrition facts label. Aim to minimize products with significant added sugars, even if naturally occurring.
- **Type of Fat:** Avoid trans fats entirely. Prioritize healthy fats from sources like nuts, seeds, and olive oil.
- **Sodium:** Many processed foods are loaded with salt. Look for options with lower sodium content.
- **Fiber:** A sign of whole-food ingredients. Higher fiber content generally means a healthier product.

The Takeaway: The food industry puts profit before our well-being. To truly understand what you're putting into your body, look beyond misleading labels and focus on ingredients and overall nutritional value.

Chapter 2: The Detox Plan – Resetting Your Body for Optimal Health

The modern world bombards us with toxins lurking in our food, environment, and even personal care products. While our bodies have natural detoxification systems, they can become overburdened. This chapter provides you with a roadmap for a tailored detox plan, designed to give your body a much-needed reset and equip you with tools to support long-term health.

Section 1: The Elimination Phase – A Time for Discovery

The first step of our detox plan involves a temporary but strategic elimination of foods commonly implicated in triggering inflammation and digestive issues. By removing these for 2-4 weeks, you'll gain clarity on how specific foods impact your well-being, empowering you to create a truly personalized, healthy eating plan. Common elimination targets include:

- Grains (even whole grains)
- Dairy
- Soy
- Processed foods
- Alcohol

· Added sugars

This elimination phase isn't merely about restriction; it's an opportunity to identify your unique food sensitivities. We'll discuss mindful reintroduction strategies, where you'll slowly add back potential trigger foods one at a time, monitoring your body's response.

Section 2: Hydration – Beyond the Basics

Water is the lifeblood of proper detoxification. However, during a detox, your needs may be greater, and understanding electrolyte balance is crucial. We'll delve into personalized water intake recommendations and how to replenish electrolytes naturally for optimal detox support. You'll also learn about other hydrating beverages, such as herbal teas and fruit-infused water, for variety and added benefits.

Section 3: Natural Detox Support – Fueling Your Body's Inner Power

This section focuses on harnessing the power of whole foods and gentle practices to bolster your body's natural detoxification pathways. We'll explore:

· Liver-Supporting Foods: We'll discuss specific fruits, vegetables, and leafy greens that act as natural cleansers for your body's primary detox organ.
· Herbs and Supplements: We'll cover potential herbs and supplements like milk thistle and dandelion root (including a vital disclaimer about consulting your healthcare provider before use).
· Gentle Practices: Learn how light exercise, sauna use, and stress management techniques aid the detoxification process.

Important Note: A detox plan should always be approached with proper guidance. Be sure to consult your healthcare provider, especially if you have any existing medical conditions.

Get ready to embark on a transformative journey. This detox plan will help you break free from food sensitivities, reduce inflammation, and unlock a new level of vibrant health and energy.

Section 1: The Elimination Phase – A Path to Personalized Nutrition

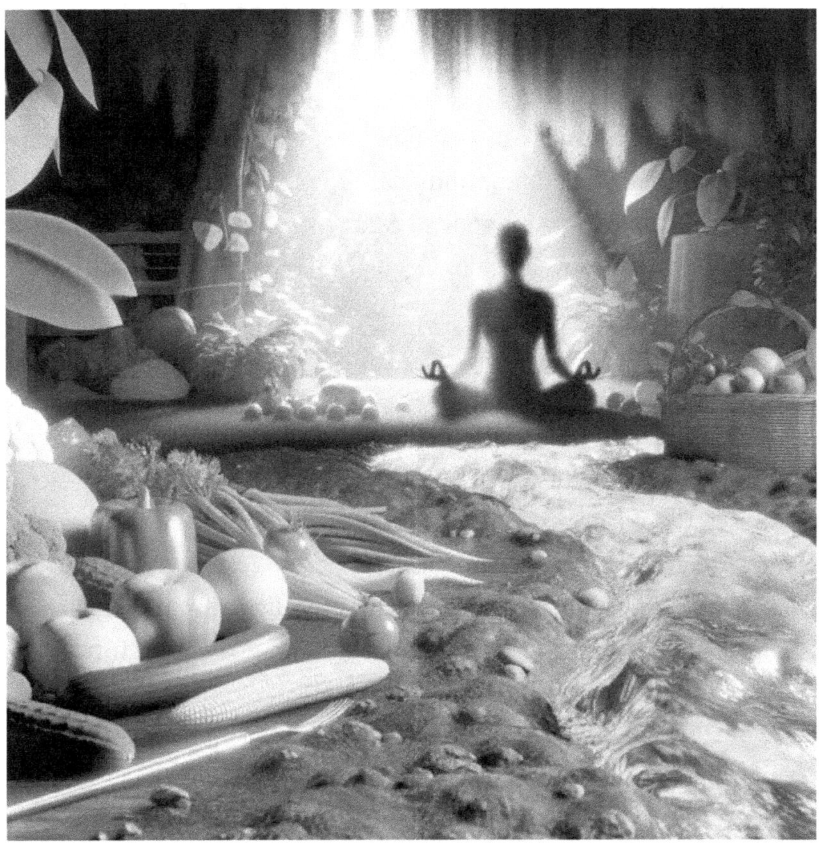

The elimination phase is a foundational step of your detox journey. It's a powerful tool that helps you understand the unique relationship between your body and the foods you eat. Let's break down the key components:

Purpose: Identifying Sensitivities and Reducing Inflammation

- **Unmasking Hidden Culprits:** Many people unknowingly live with sensitivities to common foods. These sensitivities can manifest in various ways, from digestive troubles (bloating, gas, constipation) to skin issues, headaches, fatigue, or joint pain. The elimination phase provides a "clean slate" to observe how your body functions without potential triggers.

- **Taming Inflammation:** Our modern diets often fuel chronic inflammation. The elimination phase removes major inflammatory culprits, allowing your body to calm down, repair itself, and pave the way for improved health.

Common Elimination Targets

- **Grains:** Even whole grains can temporarily irritate the gut lining in some individuals, contributing to inflammation and digestive upset. Gluten, a protein found in wheat, rye, and barley, is a common trigger for sensitivities and intolerances.
- **Dairy:** Lactose intolerance, a difficulty digesting milk sugar, is widespread. Additionally, dairy products might worsen inflammation in some people.
- **Soy:** Soy is found in a vast array of processed foods and can be an underlying allergen or digestive irritant.
- **Processed Foods:** We've already discussed the dangers lurking in processed foods – additives, artificial ingredients, refined sugars, and unhealthy fats. The elimination phase offers a clean break.
- **Alcohol:** Alcohol taxes the liver, your primary detoxification organ, and impairs its function. Giving your liver a break is essential during a detox.
- **Added Sugars:** Excessive sugar intake is a major driver of inflammation and undermines overall health.

Duration: Typically 2-4 weeks

- This period allows sufficient time to reset your system and observe noticeable improvements in your well-being. However, some individuals might benefit from slightly shorter or longer elimination protocols.

Reintroduction: Mindful Reintroduction Strategies (one food at a time)

- The Reintroduction Phase is equally crucial. After the elimination, you'll systematically reintroduce one food at a time, carefully monitoring your body's reactions.
- Keeping a detailed food and symptom journal is essential to identify which foods work well for you and those that may cause problems.

Key Takeaways:

- **The elimination phase isn't a long-term diet; it's a diagnostic tool.** It helps pinpoint trigger foods, giving you the information to create a truly personalized eating plan.
- **Prepare and commit.** Successful elimination requires planning and dedication. Stock your pantry with whole, unprocessed foods, and enlist support from family or friends.
- **Listen to your body.** Pay attention to subtle changes in how you feel both during and after the elimination phase. This knowledge is invaluable for your continued health journey.

Section 2: Hydration – The Essential Flow for Detoxification

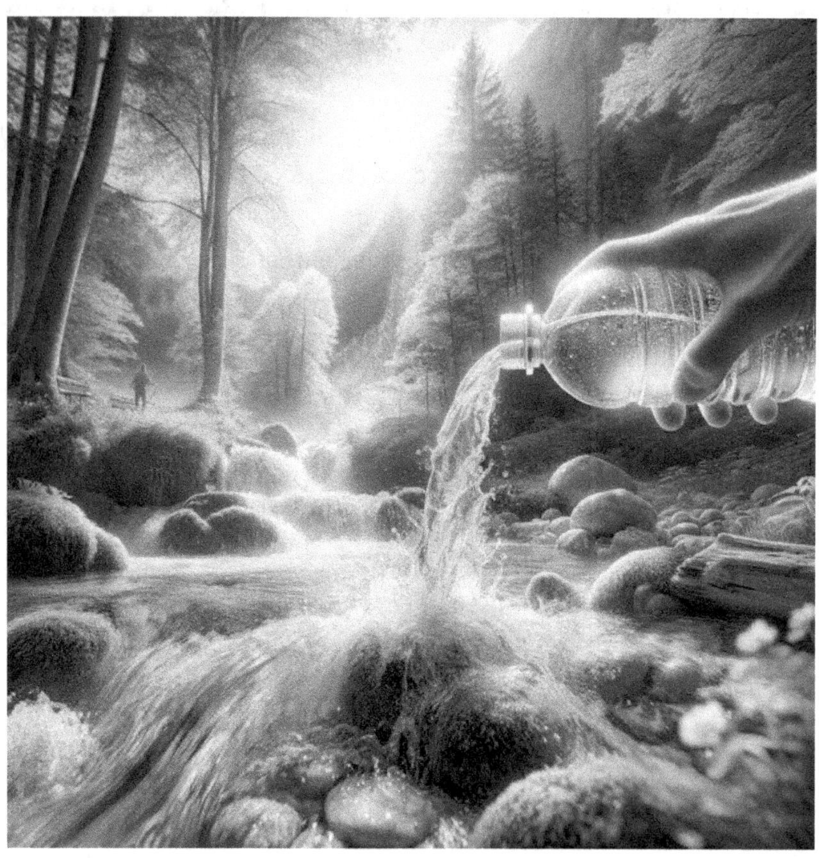

Water is vital for every bodily function, and when you're actively detoxing, maintaining optimal hydration is even more crucial. Let's explore why water is your best ally and how to ensure you're getting enough for maximized benefits.

Water Intake Recommendations: Beyond the "8 Glasses" Rule

- The classic recommendation of "8 glasses a day" is a good starting point, but your individual needs may vary. Here's how to personalize it:
- **Listen to Your Body:** Thirst is the most obvious indicator, but don't wait until you feel parched. Urine color is helpful: aim for a pale yellow.
- **Factors that Increase Needs:** Activity level, hot weather, pregnancy, breastfeeding, and certain health conditions all demand more water.
- **Calculating a Baseline:** A general guideline is half your body weight (in pounds) in ounces of water per day. Example: A 150-pound person might aim for 75 ounces (about nine 8-oz glasses) as their baseline. Adjust from there based on your individual needs.

Electrolyte Importance (Especially During Detox)

- Electrolytes are minerals that carry an electrical charge and are vital for fluid balance, nerve function, muscle contraction, and more.
- Why They Matter During Detox: Your body releases stored toxins as you detoxify, and with them, you can lose electrolytes. Imbalances can lead to headaches, fatigue, muscle cramps, and dizziness.
- How to Maintain Balance:
- **Hydrate with electrolyte-rich foods:** Leafy greens, bananas, avocados, coconut water, and bone broth are excellent natural sources.
- **Add a pinch of salt:** A tiny bit of high-quality sea salt or Himalayan salt in your water can replenish sodium, your primary electrolyte.
- **Consider Electrolyte Supplements:** For an extra boost, choose options without added sugars or artificial ingredients. Consult with your healthcare provider, especially if you have kidney or heart health issues.

- **Other Hydrating Fluids: Teas, Fruit-Infused Water**
- Variety is key to staying hydrated. Explore diverse options:
- **Herbal Teas:** Choose caffeine-free varieties like chamomile, peppermint, or ginger for their calming and digestive benefits.
- **Fruit-infused Water:** Add slices of citrus, berries, cucumber, or herbs to plain water for a refreshing flavor boost and a dose of antioxidants.

Key Takeaways:

- Consistent hydration is essential for effective detoxification. It supports your kidneys, liver, and other organs involved in toxin elimination.
- Be mindful of electrolytes, especially if you're sweating more during detox, have persistent gastrointestinal symptoms, or have underlying health conditions.
- Don't underestimate the power of plain water as your primary source of hydration. Add variety with other naturally hydrating options.

Section 3: Natural Detox Support – Harnessing the Power of Nature

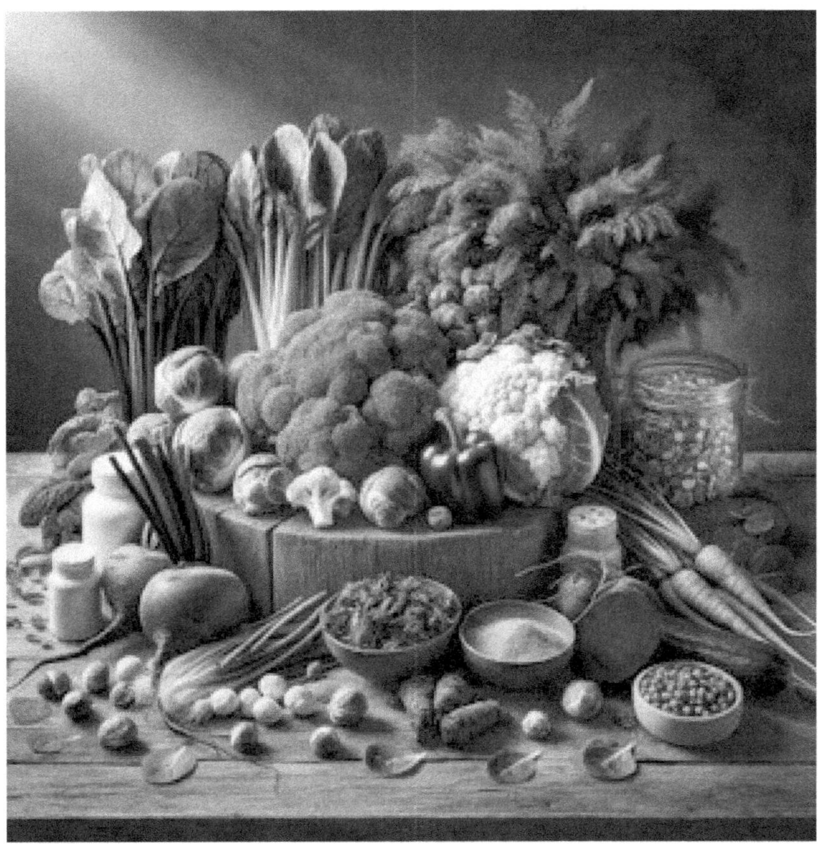

Your body has innate detoxification systems, and with the right nourishment, you can boost their efficiency. This section focuses on foods, herbs, and practices that gently support your organs of detoxification, especially your hardworking liver.

Liver-Supporting Foods: Nature's Cleansing Agents

- **Beets:** These vibrant root vegetables contain compounds called betalains, which help protect liver cells and promote bile flow, crucial for the elimination of toxins.

- **Cruciferous Vegetables:** Broccoli, cauliflower, Brussels sprouts, kale, and their relatives contain sulforaphane, a potent compound that enhances liver detoxification enzymes.
- **Leafy Greens:** Dark leafy greens like spinach, arugula, and dandelion greens are rich in chlorophyll, antioxidants, and vitamins that support liver function and overall detoxification.

Herbs and Supplements: Boosting Detoxification Pathways

- **Milk Thistle:** This herb contains silymarin, a compound with antioxidant and liver-protective properties. Studies suggest it may improve liver function and reduce inflammation.
- **Dandelion Root:** Traditionally used as a diuretic and liver tonic, dandelion root stimulates bile production, aids in toxin removal, and supports healthy digestion.

Important Disclaimer: While these herbs and supplements can be beneficial, it's crucial to consult with your healthcare provider before starting them. They may interact with certain medications or be contraindicated for specific health conditions.

Detoxifying Practices: Beyond Nutrition

- **Gentle Sweating:** Infrared saunas or light to moderate exercise can help eliminate toxins from your skin. Ensure you replenish fluids and electrolytes afterward.
- **Stress Management:** Chronic stress burdens the liver and hinders detoxification. Incorporate activities like yoga, meditation, deep breathing, or spending time in nature to mitigate stress and support overall well-being.

Key Takeaways:

- **Food as Medicine** Prioritize a diet rich in whole, plant-based foods. Their abundance of nutrients, antioxidants, and fiber naturally supports your body's detox pathways.
- **Herbs and Supplements as a Complement** They can offer additional support but shouldn't replace whole foods as your primary source of nourishment. Always seek appropriate guidance from a qualified healthcare professional.
- **Holistic Approach** Nutrition alone isn't the whole picture. Managing everyday stress and encouraging healthy detoxification through movement and sweating further amplify your body's natural processes.

Chapter 3: The Maintenance Plan – Nourishing Your Body for Lifelong Health

You've successfully navigated the detox phase, gaining invaluable insights about your body and its unique relationship with food. Now, it's time to translate that knowledge into a sustainable, nourishing eating plan that supports your health for the long term. This chapter is your guide to building a joyful and balanced approach to food, where whole,unprocessed ingredients once again take center stage.

Section 1: Embracing Whole Foods – Nature's Bounty

Let's explore the cornerstones of a health-promoting diet, emphasizing the abundance and diversity that whole foods offer:

- **Vegetables: A Rainbow of Nutrients:** Aim to fill half your plate with a variety of colorful vegetables. Experiment with different plant families and preparation methods for maximum benefits and enjoyment.
- **Fruits: Whole vs. Juice:** Prioritize whole fruits for their fiber content and blood sugar balance. While juices offer some nutrients, they lack fiber and can spike blood sugar if consumed in excess.
- **Protein: Beyond Meat:** Choose lean meats if you include them, but diversify your protein with beans, lentils, tofu,fish, and other quality

sources.

- **Healthy Fats: Essential for Well-Being:** Enjoy avocados, nuts, seeds, olive oil, and other sources of healthy fats in moderation. These are beneficial for heart health, satiety, and nutrient absorption.
- **Whole Grains: Proceed with Caution:** If tolerated, focus on true whole grains with a high grain-to-fiber ratio (like quinoa, oats). Experiment and see how your body responds.

Section 2: Meal Planning and Practicality – Making Nourishment Work for You

Healthy eating doesn't need to be complicated. Let's discuss strategies that fit seamlessly into your lifestyle:

- **Batch Cooking and Prep:** Dedicate some time on the weekend to pre-chop vegetables, roast a medley, or cook a big pot of soup or beans for convenient grab-and-go meals.
- **Smart Snacking:** Have healthy snacks like cut-up veggies, fruits, yogurt, or nuts on hand to prevent energy crashes and unhealthy cravings.
- **Quick, Balanced Meals:** Develop a repertoire of simple recipes focusing on whole foods that come together quickly for busy weeknights.

Section 3: Portion Control and Mindful Eating – Reconnecting Body and Mind

This section focuses on building a healthy relationship with food, rooted in mindful awareness instead of strict limitations.

- **Portion Guides:** Use your hand as a rough guide, alongside visual cues from trusted resources, to help you estimate appropriate portions without obsessive calorie counting.

- **Tuning In:** Practice slowing down, paying attention to your body's hunger, fullness, and enjoyment signals. Put down the fork between bites, chew thoroughly, and savor your food.
- **Intuitive Eating:** We'll discuss the principles of intuitive eating, learning to trust your body's innate wisdom and let go of rigid diet rules.

Key Takeaway: Nourishing your body is an act of self-love. Sustainable healthy eating shouldn't feel restrictive or overly complicated. This chapter provides a practical roadmap to make delicious, whole-food choices a joyful and enduring part of your life.

Section 1: Embracing Whole Foods – Building Blocks for Optimal Health

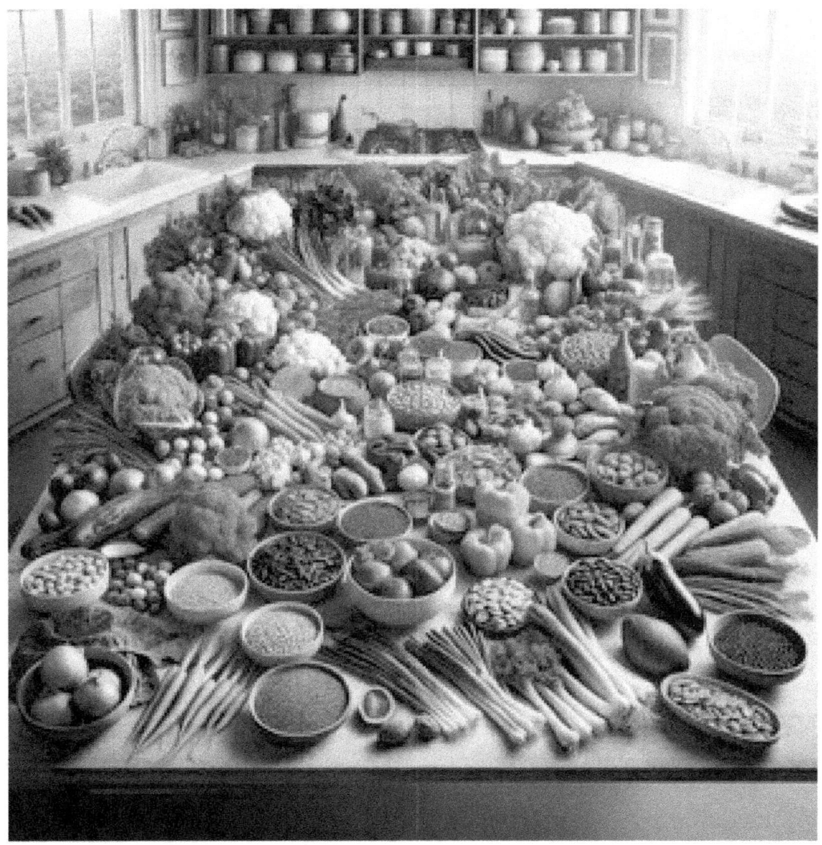

By prioritizing whole foods, you provide your body with the rich array of nutrients it needs to thrive. In this section, we'll delve into the diverse world of whole-food options, exploring how they work synergistically to support your long-term health and well-being.

Vegetables: Variety is Key, Emphasizing Different Colors and Plant Families

- **The Power of the Rainbow:** Aim to eat a wide range of colorful vegetables daily. Different pigments signal different phytonutrients – powerful plant compounds with antioxidant and anti-inflammatory benefits.

- **Plant Families:** Don't just stick to carrots and broccoli. Branch out with:
- Cruciferous: Broccoli, kale, cauliflower, Brussels sprouts.
- Leafy Greens: Spinach, arugula, Swiss chard, collard greens.
- Allium Family: Garlic, onions, leeks, scallions.
- Nightshades: Tomatoes, bell peppers, eggplant.
- Root Vegetables: Beets, carrots, sweet potatoes, parsnips.

Fruits: Whole Fruits vs. Juices, Blood Sugar Considerations

- **Fiber is Your Friend:** Whole fruits provide fiber, which slows down the release of sugar into your bloodstream, promoting stable blood sugar levels. Juices lack this fiber, causing faster, more dramatic spikes.
- **Enjoy in Moderation:** While rich in vitamins and antioxidants, fruits still contain natural sugars. Pair with protein or healthy fat for sustained energy and balanced blood sugar response. Think apple slices with almond butter or berries with plain Greek yogurt.

Protein: Diverse Sources (beans, lentils, tofu, fish, lean meats)

- **Plant-Based Powerhouses:** Beans, lentils, and tofu are excellent sources of protein, fiber, and essential nutrients. They're also incredibly versatile in cooking.
- **Fish: Focus on Fatty Varieties**: Salmon, sardines, and mackerel offer protein and beneficial omega-3 fatty acids crucial for heart health, brain function, and reducing inflammation.
- **Lean Meats (if included):** Opt for skinless chicken, turkey, lean

grass-fed beef, or pork in moderation, prioritizing other protein sources first.

Healthy Fats: Oils, Nuts, Seeds, Avocados

- **Essential for Well-being:** Healthy fats are vital for nutrient absorption, satiety, hormone balance, and overall health.
- **Choose Wisely:**
- Oils: Emphasize extra virgin olive oil, avocado oil, and other unrefined oils.
- Nuts and Seeds: Go for almonds, walnuts, pumpkin seeds, chia seeds, and flaxseeds – each with a unique nutritional profile.
- Avocados: A creamy, delicious source of fiber, potassium, and healthy monounsaturated fats.

Whole Grains: Only if Tolerated, Maximizing the Grain-to-Fiber Ratio

- **Individual Considerations:** Some people thrive on whole grains, while others experience digestive discomfort. Proceed based on your body's response during the elimination phase.
- **Smart Choices (if tolerated):** Prioritize grains with a high grain-to-fiber ratio, like:
- Quinoa
- Oats (rolled or steel-cut)
- Brown Rice
- Buckwheat
- Amaranth

Key Takeaway: Embracing whole foods nourishes your body at the cellular level, providing the building blocks for optimal health, energy, and disease prevention. Let their colors, textures, and flavors be your guide as you create vibrant, delicious, and deeply satisfying meals.

Section 2: Meal Planning and Practicality – Integrating Healthy Eating into Your Lifestyle

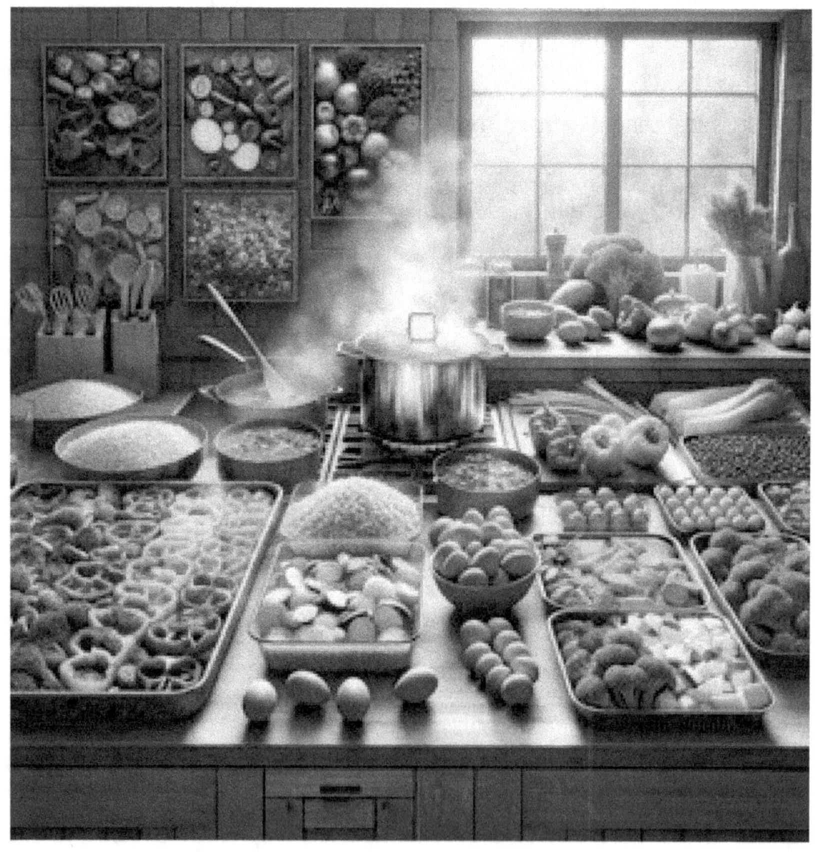

Maintaining a nourishing diet long-term requires a smart approach.

This section focuses on strategies that help you effortlessly incorporate whole-food meals into your busy life, making healthy eating a sustainable and enjoyable habit.

Batch Cooking and Weekly Prep Strategies

- **Your Time-Saving Superpower:** Dedicate a few hours on the weekend to pre-prep ingredients for the week ahead. This sets you up for success with healthy options readily available.
- **Examples:**
- Roast a big tray of vegetables (peppers, onions, broccoli, sweet potatoes, etc.)
- Cook a pot of quinoa, brown rice, or lentils.
- Hard-boil several eggs for easy protein.
- Wash and chop fruits and vegetables for snacks or quick salads.
- Make a double batch of soup or stew for lunches or dinners.

Healthy Snacking for Sustained Energy

- **Prevent Hunger-Driven Choices:** Having healthy snacks on hand is essential to maintain consistent energy and prevent cravings for unhealthy options.
- **Smart Snack Ideas:**
- Fruit + Nuts or Seeds: Apple slices with almond butter, and pear with a handful of walnuts.
- Veggies + Dip: Carrots and hummus, celery sticks with guacamole.
- Plain Greek Yogurt + Berries: Provides protein, probiotics, and antioxidants.
- Hard-boiled Egg + Whole Grain Crackers: Simple and satisfying.
- Homemade Trail Mix: Combine nuts, seeds, and a bit of unsweetened dried fruit.

Quick, Balanced Meal Ideas

- **Healthy Doesn't Mean Complicated:** Focus on combining key food groups for satisfying meals that come together quickly. Here are a few ideas:
- **Protein + Veggies + Whole Grain:** Grilled chicken breast with roasted vegetables and quinoa.
- **Salad Power Bowls:** Start with a bed of leafy greens, add roasted chickpeas, avocado, cucumber, tomatoes, a drizzle of olive oil, and balsamic vinegar.
- **Eggs for Any Meal:** Scrambled eggs with sautéed spinach and whole-grain toast, or a veggie frittata.
- **Leftover Reinvention:** Turn leftover roasted chicken into a whole wheat wrap with lettuce and mustard or cooked quinoa into a Buddha bowl with avocado and roasted vegetables.

Key Takeaways:

- **Planning is key.** A little effort upfront saves time and stress during the week, making it easier to stick to your healthy eating plan.
- **Keep it simple.** Don't overcomplicate meals. A few whole-food ingredients can combine into countless delicious and nutritious options.
- **Listen to Your Body** There are days when you'll have more time for cooking and others when you need quick solutions. Both can fit into this healthy eating plan.

Section 3: Portion Control & Mindful Eating – Reconnecting with Your Body's Wisdom

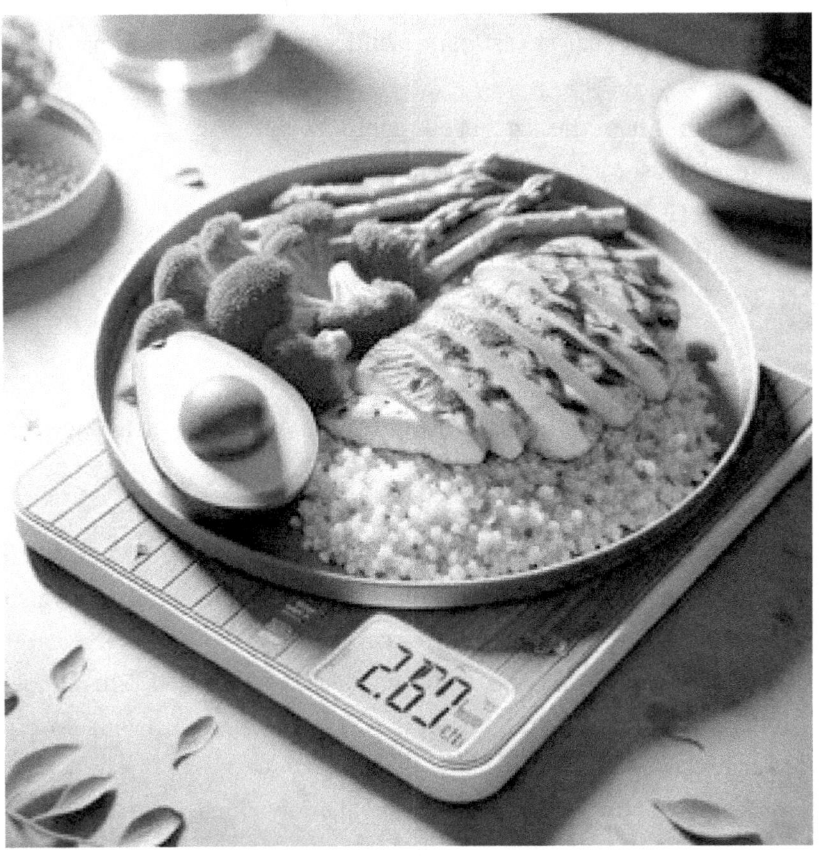

True nourishment goes beyond what's on your plate. This section empowers you to tune into your body's signals, creating a more intuitive and sustainable way of eating that supports both your physical and emotional well-being.

Visual Portion Guides vs. Counting Calories

- **The Problem with Calories:** Focusing solely on calorie counting can be misleading and unsustainable. Not all calories are created equal – nutrient density matters more for health and satiety.
- **Visual Cues:** Learn to estimate healthy portions using simple visual guides:
- Protein: About the size of your palm.
- Vegetables: Aim to fill half your plate.
- Whole Grains (if included): About a cupped handful.
- Healthy Fats: A serving is around the size of your thumb.
- **The Hand as a Tool** Your hand size is roughly proportionate to your body size, making it a personalized portion guide.

Techniques for Slowing Down: Putting Down the Fork, Chewing Thoroughly

- **Rushing Hinders Digestion:** Eating quickly prevents you from registering fullness cues, leading to potential overeating. It also compromises your digestion process.
- **Put the Fork Down:** Place your fork down between bites. This simple act introduces a pause, allowing you to check in with your satiety levels.
- **Chew Well:** Chewing thoroughly breaks down food, aiding digestion and nutrient absorption. It also enhances the flavor and enjoyment of your meal. Aim for 20-30 chews per bite.

Intuitive Eating Principles: Recognizing Hunger and Fullness Cues

- **Diet Culture Disconnect:** Constant dieting and external rules can leave us out of touch with our natural hunger and satiety signals.

- **Tuning In:** Intuitive eating helps you rebuild trust in your body. Start paying attention to:
- Physical Hunger: Gurgling stomach, low energy, slight lightheadedness.
- Gentle Fullness: A comfortable feeling of satisfaction, no longer feeling the urge to keep eating.
- Overfullness: Bloating, sluggishness, discomfort.
- **The Hunger Scale:** Many resources exist online to help you identify your level of hunger and fullness on a scale of 1-10.

Key Takeaways

- **Ditch the Diet Mentality** Release yourself from rigid rules and obsessive calorie counting.
- **Mindful eating fosters a healthier relationship with food.** It teaches you to listen to your body's internal cues, promoting balance and enjoyment.
- **Be Patient:** Relearning to trust your body takes time and practice. Be kind to yourself throughout this process.

Chapter 4: Food for Life – Finding Freedom and Lasting Balance

We've now equipped you with the tools to make informed food choices that nourish your body. Yet, our relationship with food extends far beyond physical needs. This chapter delves into the emotional side of eating, helping you break free from unhealthy patterns and forge a sustainable, joyful, and empowering relationship with food.

Section 1: Emotional Eating and Mindful Solutions

Food often becomes intertwined with our emotions, providing temporary comfort or distraction. Let's unpack the connection between food and mood:

- **Triggers:** We'll identify common triggers for emotional eating, such as stress, boredom, sadness, or difficult life events.
- **Finding Alternatives:** Instead of automatically reaching for food when emotions strike, we'll explore healthier coping mechanisms. Techniques like journaling, mindful walks, or finding non-food rewards can be powerful tools.
- **Addressing the Root Cause:** Ultimately, working with underlying emotions, through therapy or other professional support if needed, is key to breaking free from the cycle of emotional eating.

Section 2: Building Sustainable Habits

Sustainable healthy eating isn't about overnight perfection. Let's ditch the harmful "all or nothing" mentality that sets us up for failure.

- **Small, Gradual Shifts:** Focus on small, achievable changes. Start by adding a colorful vegetable to your meals or swapping sugary drinks for water most days of the week.
- **Joyful Exploration:** Reframe healthy living as an exciting adventure. Explore farmers' markets, experiment with new recipes using whole ingredients, and discover the simple pleasure of cooking for yourself.
- **Progress, Not Perfection:** Embrace the ups and downs of this journey. Celebrate every success, and allow yourself compassion when faced with setbacks.

Section 3: Social Navigation

Eating out and social events don't have to derail your progress. We'll discuss:

- **Mindful Restaurant Strategies:** Learn how to navigate menus, ask the right questions about ingredients, and prioritize healthy options while still enjoying social dining experiences.
- **Travel and Events:** Explore strategies for making healthy choices on the go and during gatherings centered around food.
- **Balance and Self-Care:** We'll focus on prioritizing your health goals without feeling isolated or deprived. You can thrive in social settings while remaining true to your commitment to nourishing your body.

Key Takeaway: True food freedom comes through understanding your emotional relationship with food, developing sustainable habits, and navigating real-life social situations with confidence. Let this chapter guide you toward a healthy,balanced, and truly enjoyable connection with food that lasts a lifetime.

Section 1: Emotional Eating and Mindful Solutions – Breaking the Cycle

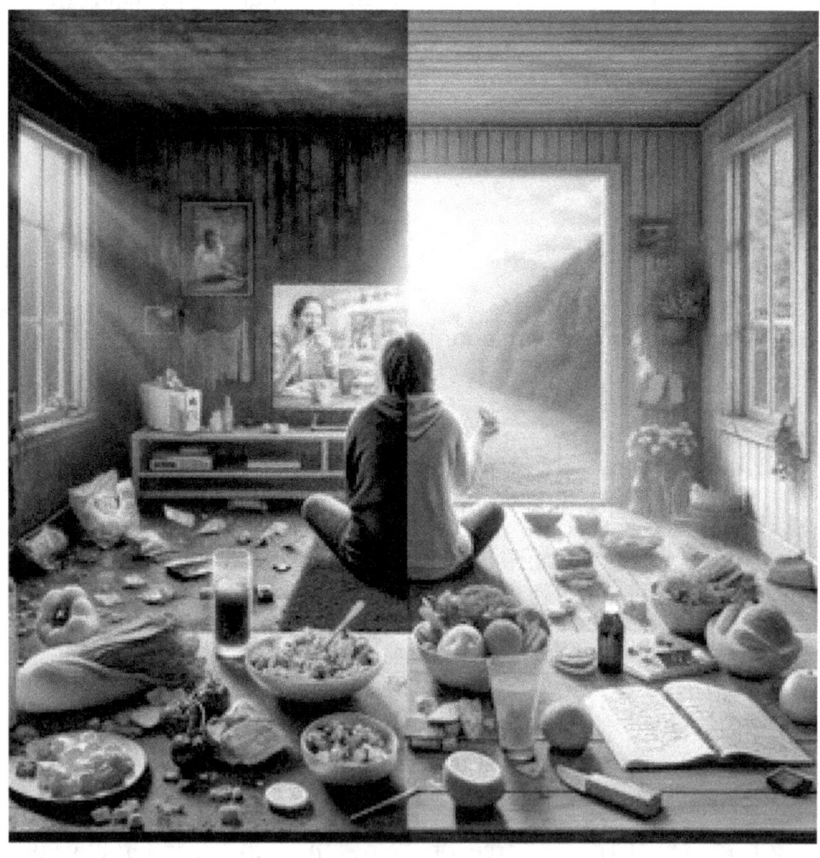

For many, food becomes a crutch for coping with uncomfortable emotions rather than simple nourishment. This section aims to illuminate the complex link between our feelings and eating habits, offering tools to break free from the cycle of emotional eating.

Understanding the Food-Mood Connection

- **Stress Response:** Chronic stress releases cortisol, causing cravings for sugary, fatty "comfort foods" that provide a temporary energy boost and a fleeting sense of reward.
- **Seeking Comfort:** Food is often used as a way to numb uncomfortable emotions like sadness, loneliness, anxiety, or boredom.
- **Learned Association**: From childhood, we may have been rewarded with treats or soothed with food, creating a deep-seated link between emotions and eating.

Identifying Your Triggers

- **Becoming a Self-Detective:** The first step towards change is understanding your unique triggers:
- Stressful workdays?
- Certain social situations?
- Feeling lonely or bored?
- **Start an "Emotional Eating Journal":** Track not only what you eat in challenging moments but also the emotions you are feeling beforehand. This awareness is key for developing alternative strategies.

Techniques: Journaling, Non-Food Rewards, Addressing Underlying Emotions

- **The Power of Journaling:** Putting your feelings down on paper can defuse their intensity and bring clarity to your eating patterns. Free-form writing or using prompts specific to emotional eating can be insightful.

- **Finding New Rewards:** When cravings hit, what non-food activities bring even a sliver of joy or relief? Examples:
- A quick walk in nature
- Listening to your favorite song
- Taking a relaxing bath
- Calling a supportive friend
- **Addressing the Root Cause** While these techniques are helpful, long-lasting change often requires tackling the underlying emotions. If emotional eating is a significant struggle, consider enlisting professional support from a therapist or counselor specializing in eating behaviors.

Key Takeaways

- **Guilt is Counterproductive:** Recognize that emotional eating is a common coping mechanism. Be kind to yourself as you work towards building healthier habits.
- **Food is just one tool:** Nourishing your body is essential, but so is nurturing your emotional well-being. Finding healthy ways to express and manage your emotions is vital for a sustainable, balanced relationship with food.
- **Seek Support:** If you're struggling, don't hesitate to reach out for help. Therapists or support groups can provide tools and guidance tailored to your individual needs.

Section 2: Building Sustainable Habits – Embracing the Journey

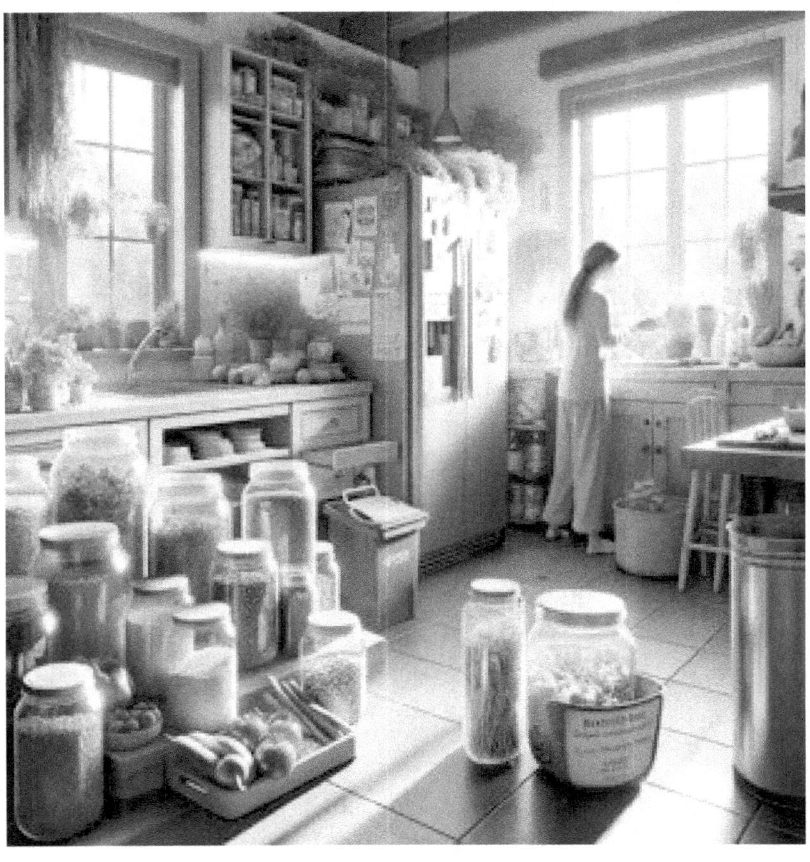

Transforming your relationship with food is a journey, not a sprint. This section empowers you to let go of rigid expectations and cultivate a positive, sustainable approach to healthy living.

The "All or Nothing" Mentality Danger

- **The Setup for Failure:** Viewing healthy eating as an all-or-nothing game sets you up to feel defeated by the slightest slip-up. One "bad" meal or day can trigger feelings of guilt and derail your progress.
- **Focus on the Big Picture:** Instead of obsessing over perfection, prioritize consistency and celebrate overall progress. Did you make healthier choices most days of the week? That's a win!

Small, Gradual Shifts

- **The Power of Tiny Changes:** Don't underestimate the impact of small, manageable adjustments. Here are some examples:
- Add one serving of vegetables to each meal.
- Swap sugary drinks for water or herbal tea most of the time.
- Start prepping one healthy snack per day.
- Try one new healthy recipe per week.
- **Celebrate Your Victories:** Acknowledge and applaud even the smallest of wins. This positive reinforcement builds momentum and reinforces your commitment.

Cultivate Joy Around Healthy Cooking and Exploration

- **Reframe Your Mindset:** Cooking shouldn't feel like a chore. Approach it with a sense of curiosity and adventure.
- **Simple and Delicious:** Start with easy-to-follow recipes emphasizing whole-food ingredients. Discover the satisfying flavors that come from nourishing your body. Seek out online resources and cookbooks dedicated to approachable, healthy cooking.
- **Farmers Market Adventures:** Explore the vibrant produce at farmers' markets or local farms. Let the seasonal bounty inspire your

culinary creations.

- **Make it Social:** Invite a friend or partner to join you in the kitchen. Cooking together adds a fun and supportive element to healthy eating.

Key Takeaways

- **Consistency over Perfection:** Long-lasting change comes from small, sustainable habits practiced consistently.
- **Progress is Personal:** Your journey is unique. Avoid comparing yourself to others, and focus on celebrating your victories.
- **Food Can Be Fun:** Approach healthy cooking and exploration with joy and curiosity. Let it become a source of creativity and enjoyment, a vital part of your self-care routine.

Section 3: Social Navigation – Maintaining Your Healthy Path

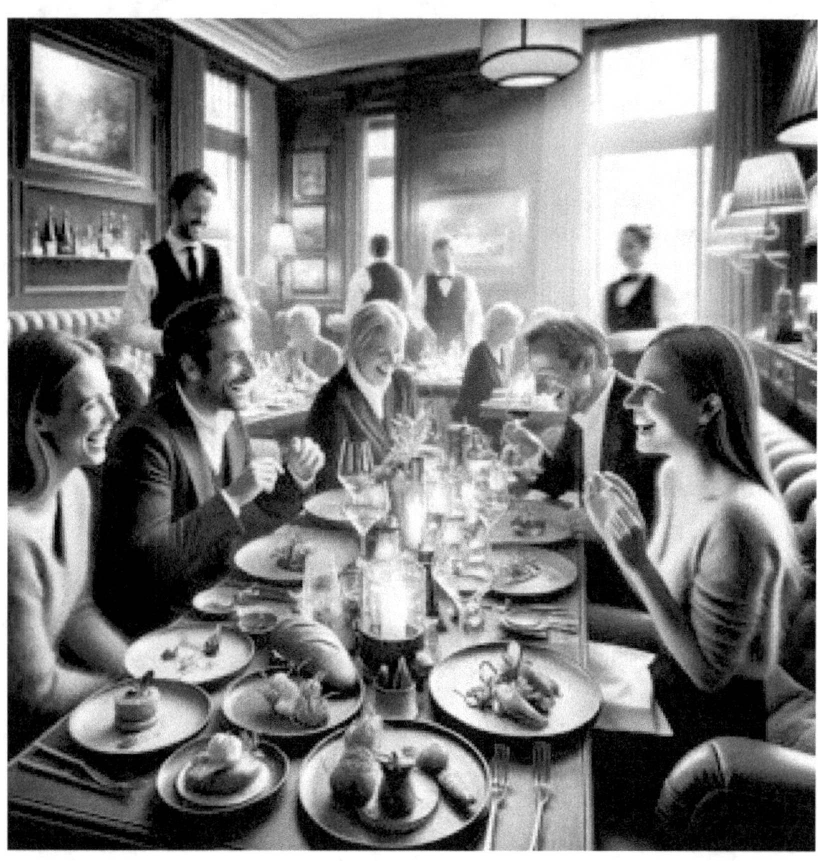

Enjoying social events and dining out shouldn't necessitate abandoning your healthy eating goals. This section empowers you with strategies to navigate social situations with confidence, prioritizing your well-being without feeling isolated or deprived.

Ordering Strategies at Restaurants

- **Pre-Scan the Menu:** Many restaurants offer online menus. Take some time beforehand to identify potentially healthier options and avoid impulsive choices based on hunger.

- **Mindful Modifications:** Don't be afraid to ask questions about ingredients, cooking methods, and request adjustments:
- Dressing on the side
- Swap fries for a side salad
- Order grilled or steamed instead of fried
- Request sauce on the side for better portion control
- **Prioritizing Whole Foods:** Seek out dishes emphasizing vegetables, lean proteins, and healthy grains (if tolerated). Be wary of dishes laden with creamy sauces, heavy breading, or overly cheesy toppings.

Preparing for Travel and Social Events

- **The Importance of Planning:** Being caught hungry and unprepared can lead to unhealthy decisions.
- **Travel Snacks:** Pack nutritious options like nuts, fruit, pre-cut veggies, or whole-grain crackers.
- **Research Your Destination:** If staying somewhere with a kitchen, explore grocery stores and healthy eateries in advance.
- **Potlucks & Gatherings:** If appropriate, offer to bring a healthy dish you enjoy to share with others. This ensures at least one reliable option.

Prioritizing Your Health Without Isolation

- **Be Confident, Not Apologetic:** Avoid feeling the need to justify your food choices. A simple "That looks delicious, but I'm going to opt for something lighter" is sufficient.
- **Focus on the Company:** Remember, social gatherings are about connecting with loved ones, not just the food. Shift your focus to

enjoying conversations and the overall experience.

- **Treats in Moderation:** It's okay to indulge occasionally. Choose a small treat you truly savor and enjoy it mindfully, guilt-free.

Key Takeaways:

- **Planning is key.** A little forethought empowers you to navigate any social occasion without compromising your health goals.
- **Don't be afraid to speak up.** Restaurants are generally willing to accommodate requests to support healthier dining.
- **It's about balance.** Healthy eating supports a joyful social life, and occasional indulgences are part of a sustainable approach.

Chapter 5: Exercise – Adding Movement to Your Routine

Important Disclaimer: Consult with your healthcare provider before embarking on any new exercise program, especially if you have any existing health conditions or are new to physical activity.

Section 1: The Benefits of Exercise – Rewards Beyond a Smaller Waistline

Exercise is a powerful tool that benefits body, mind, and spirit. Let's explore why prioritizing movement can be life-changing:

- **Weight Management: Burning Calories and Boosting Metabolism** Exercise increases calorie expenditure,supporting weight loss or a healthy weight. It also builds muscle, which burns more calories at rest than fat tissue.
- **Chronic Disease Prevention: Protecting Your Future Self** Regular exercise reduces the risk of:
- Heart disease
- Type 2 diabetes
- Certain cancers
- Stroke
- And more!

- **Mood Enhancement: Your Natural Stress-Buster** Exercise releases endorphins, our feel-good hormones,combating stress, anxiety, and boosting energy levels. It also improves sleep, another crucial pillar of well-being.
- **Cognitive Function: Maintaining Cognitive Sharpness and Focus** Studies suggest that exercise increases blood flow to the brain, protecting cognitive function and potentially reducing the risk of dementia.
- **Overall Well-being: Strength, Posture, and Longevity**
- Exercise builds strength and flexibility, improving posture and functional daily movement.
- It's an investment in your long-term healthspan, maximizing quality of life for years to come.

Section 2: Designing Your Fitness Plan

The best workout plan is the one you'll stick with! Focus on enjoyment and variety:

- **Finding Enjoyment:** Think about activities that spark a sense of joy or playfulness. Do you thrive with a workout buddy or prefer solo adventures? This discovery ensures your plan is motivating and sustainable.
- **Types of Exercise:**
- **Cardio:** Elevate that heart rate! Walking, running, swimming, cycling, dancing all count. Aim for at least 150 minutes of moderate-intensity or 75 minutes of vigorous-intensity aerobic exercise per week, spread throughout the week.
- **Strength Training:** Build stronger muscles and bones with body-weight exercises, resistance bands, or weightlifting. Aim for 2-3 sessions per week.

- **Flexibility** Improve range of motion and reduce soreness with yoga, pilates, or targeted stretches. Aim for several times a week, even for short periods.
- **Mixing it Up** Variety keeps your body challenged and your mind engaged, maximizing results and preventing boredom.

Section 3: Getting Started

- **Start Small:** No need to be a gym rat from day one! Short bursts of activity throughout the day count.
- **Gradual Progression** Listen to your body and gradually increase duration, intensity, or frequency over time.
- **Making It a Habit** Schedule exercise like any appointment. Link movement to existing routines (a walk after dinner, a morning stretch routine).
- **Setting Realistic Goals** Prioritize consistency over intensity. Celebrate the small wins that make exercise a lasting part of your life.
- **Listen to Your Body** Rest is essential for recovery and progress. Pay attention to signs of overexertion and honor your body's need for breaks.

Key Takeaway: Exercise is about feeling good, inside and out. Explore with a sense of playfulness and celebrate the incredible ways movement enhances your life. This joyful, sustainable approach is the key to long-term success.

Section 1: The Benefits of Exercise – Your Prescription for a Healthier, Happier Life

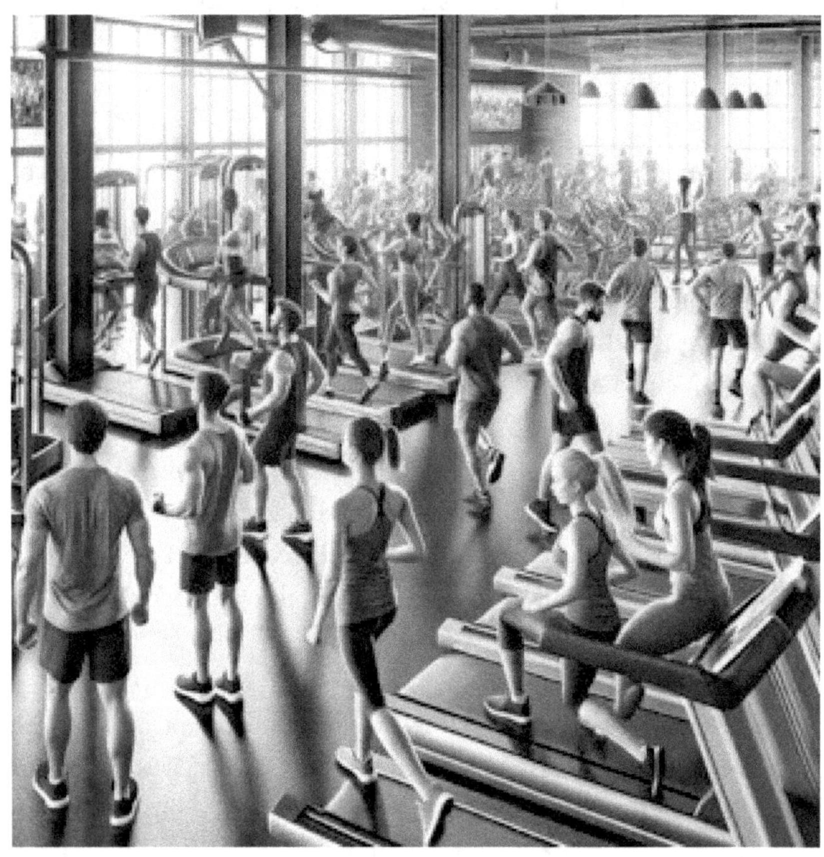

When we talk about exercise, the focus often centers on weight loss. While an excellent benefit, the transformative powers of movement extend far beyond what the scale reflects. Let's explore how regular physical activity can change your life, both inside and out.

Weight Management: Burning Calories and Boosting Metabolism

- **Burn Baby Burn:** Exercise directly burns calories, creating the deficit needed for weight loss or maintenance.
- **Muscle Power:** Building lean muscle mass elevates your resting metabolic rate. Think of your muscles as little calorie-burning engines, working for you even when you're at rest.

Chronic Disease Prevention: Shielding Your Future Self

- **Heart Healthy:** Exercise strengthens your heart, lowers blood pressure, and improves cholesterol levels, slashing your risk of heart disease.
- **Diabetes Defense:** Exercise improves insulin sensitivity, helping to regulate blood sugar levels and reducing your risk for type 2 diabetes, or better managing it if already diagnosed.
- **Beyond the Big Two:** Exercise offers protective benefits against a host of other chronic conditions, including certain cancers, osteoporosis, stroke, and more.

Mood Enhancement: Your Natural Stress-Buster and Energizer

- **Endorphin Rush:** Exercise triggers the release of endorphins, our body's mood-boosting chemicals, reducing anxiety and promoting a sense of well-being.
- **Sound Sleep:** Regular physical activity improves sleep quality, essential for emotional and physical health.
- **Busting Fatigue:** Intuitively, you might think exercise will tire you out, but the opposite is true! It combats fatigue and boosts energy levels long-term.

Cognitive Function: Maintaining Cognitive Sharpness and Focus

- **Brain Booster:** Research suggests exercise increases blood flow to the brain, improving memory, and focus, and protecting against age-related cognitive decline.
- **Mental Clarity:** Physical activity can alleviate "brain fog" and boost mental alertness to tackle your daily tasks.

Overall Well-being: Strength, Posture, and Longevity

- **Feeling Strong:** Exercise builds muscle strength, making everyday activities easier, reducing injury risk, and giving you a sense of empowerment.
- **Standing Tall:** Regular movement, especially exercises targeted for core and back muscles, improves posture, helping you look and feel more confident.
- **Invest in Longevity:** Exercise isn't just about adding years to your life, but truly adding LIFE to your years. It combats frailty and age-related declines, maximizing your ability to live a vibrant, independent life.

Key Takeaway: Think of exercise as a potent form of preventive medicine. It's a wise investment in your physical, mental, and emotional well-being, both now and for the years to come.

Section 2: Designing Your Fitness Plan – Discover the Joy of Movement

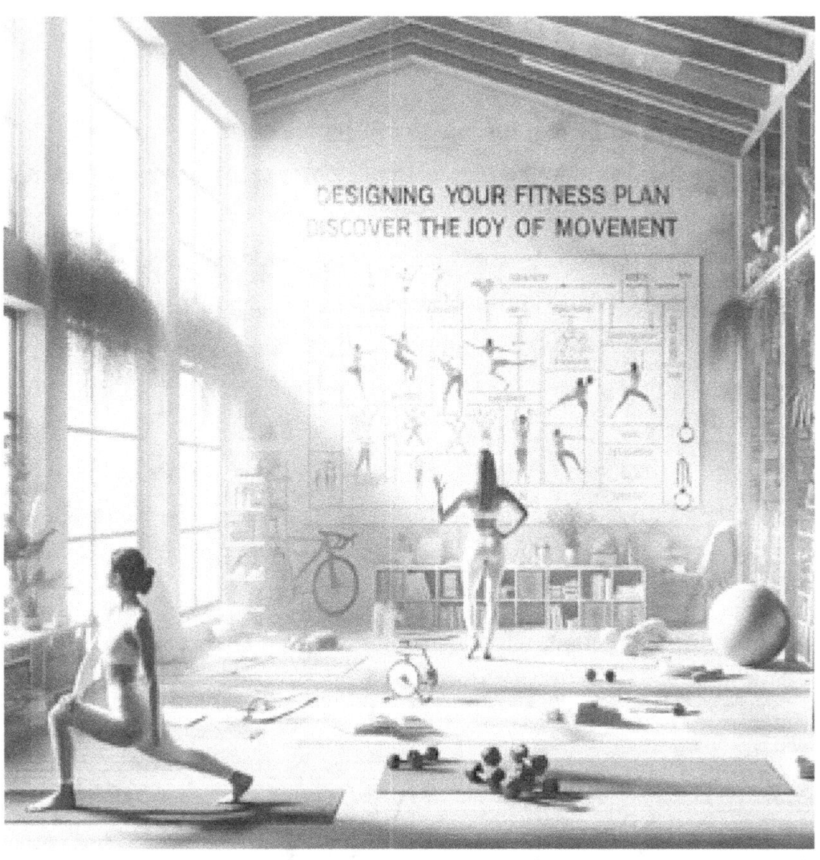

The best exercise plan is the one you enjoy and stick with long-term. This section helps you build a routine that's not only effective but sparks a sense of excitement and nourishes your well-being holistically.

Finding Enjoyment: Prioritize Activities that are Intrinsically Fun and Motivating

- **The Importance of Play:** Think back to childhood – did you love playing tag, riding bikes, or dancing to your favorite songs? Exercise shouldn't feel like a chore; tap into that inner sense of joy and playfulness.
- **Exploration and Curiosity:** Don't be afraid to experiment! Try different classes, join a recreational sports team, or explore nature trails – you might surprise yourself and find a new passion.
- **Social Connection:** If working out with a buddy or group motivates you, embrace that! Find workout partners or group fitness classes that create a sense of community.

Types of Exercise

Cardio (Walking, Running, Swimming, Dancing): Get That Heart Pumping!

- **Benefits:** Improves cardiovascular health, burns calories, boosts mood.
- **Variety is Key:** Spice it up with hiking, dancing, swimming, cycling – find what energizes you!

Strength Training (Bodyweight Exercises, Weightlifting, Resistance Bands): Build Strong Foundations

- **Benefits:** Builds muscle, improves posture, supports weight management, protects bone health.
- **Progression:** Start with bodyweight exercises (squats, lunges, push-ups) and gradually progress to weights or resistance bands, if

desired.

Flexibility (Yoga, Pilates, Stretching): Enhance Range of Motion and Reduce Soreness

- **Benefits:** Improves flexibility, reduces muscle tension, complements other workouts, and promotes mind-body connection.
- **Tailor it:** Choose yoga styles that fit your goals – from gentle restorative to dynamic, strength-building flows.

Mixing it Up: Variety Improves Results and Prevents Boredom

- **Challenge Your Body:** Alternating types of exercise prevent plateaus and maximize results. Your body adapts quickly, and variety keeps it challenged.
- **Beat Burnout:** Boredom is a major reason people abandon exercise. Switching things up keeps it fresh and engaging.
- **Sample Plan Example:** Try this as a starting point, adjusting to your preferences:
- Monday: Strength training
- Tuesday: Cardio (brisk walking, dancing)
- Wednesday: Rest or gentle yoga
- Thursday: Strength training (different focus than Monday)
- Friday: Cardio (swimming, cycling)
- Weekend: Active fun (hiking, outdoor play)

Key Takeaways:

- **Listen to Your Body:** What feels good? What sparks a sense of excitement? Use these internal cues to guide your plan.
- **Find Your Tribe:** If the community motivates you, discover the

power of working out with like-minded individuals.

- **Evolve Your Routine:** As your fitness improves, adjust your plan to stay challenged. Keep the joy of movement alive!

Section 3: Getting Started – Your Journey to a More Active Life

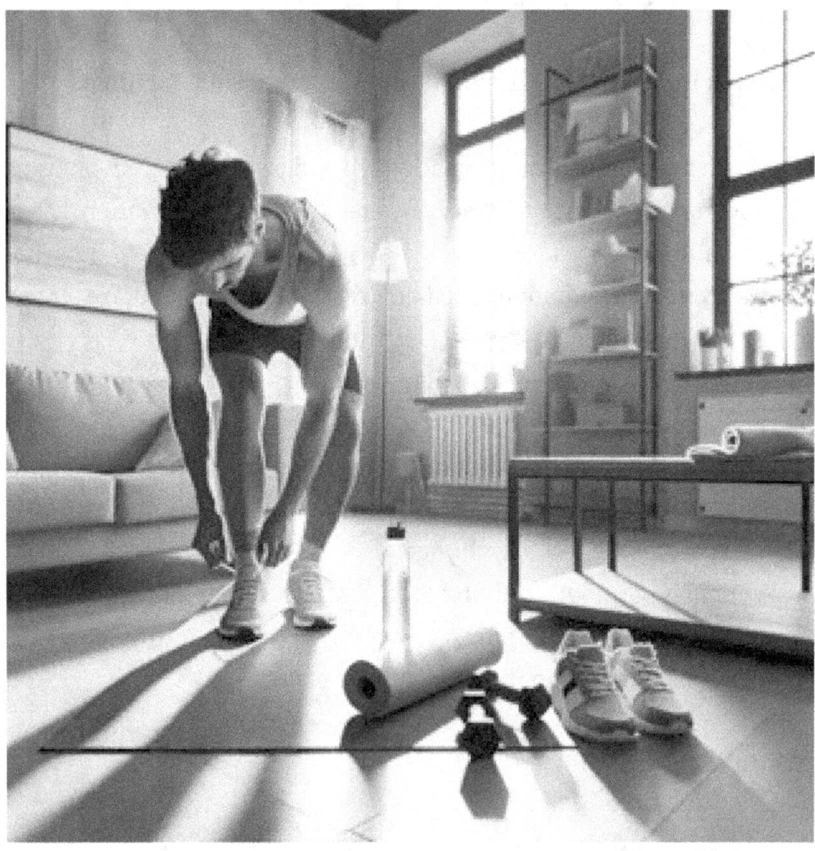

Starting a new exercise routine can feel daunting, but remember, every journey begins with a single step. This section focuses on strategies that set you up for success, making fitness an empowering and joyful part of your life.

Start Small: Short, Manageable Bursts of Activity

- **Don't Overwhelm Yourself:** Trying to do too much, too soon is a recipe for burnout. Begin with short bursts of movement throughout the day.
- **Examples:**
- 10-minute walks during breaks
- Taking stairs instead of the elevator
- A quick bodyweight workout while watching TV

Gradual Progression: Increasing Frequency, Duration, or Intensity Over Time

- **Slow and Steady Wins:** Avoid injury and improve your chances of sticking with the plan by gradually increasing exercise difficulty over time.
- **Ways to Progress:**
- Add a few minutes to your walks each week.
- Gradually increase the number of reps or sets in strength workouts.
- Try a slightly faster pace or incline during cardio sessions.

Making It a Habit: Building Movement into Your Daily Routine

- **Consistency is Key:** Short, frequent workouts are often more sustainable than long sessions you dread and eventually skip.
- **Link it Up:** Attach movement to existing habits. Walk while listening

to your favorite podcast, do stretches during your morning coffee ritual, or have a dance break while cooking.

- **Schedule it:** Treat workouts like non-negotiable appointments. Putting them in your calendar increases the likelihood of following through.

Setting Realistic Goals: Focus on Consistency and Enjoyment

- **Beyond Aesthetics:** Shift your focus from weight loss alone to how exercise makes you FEEL. Celebrate increased energy, improved mood, and a sense of accomplishment.
- **Progress, not Perfection:** Prioritize consistency over intensity. Did you move your body most days of the week? That's a win to be proud of!

Listening to Your Body: Balance Ambition with Respecting Your Limits

- **Rest is Essential:** Schedule rest days into your plan! This allows your body to recover and rebuild, preventing injury.
- **Know the Difference:** Good soreness is different from pain. If something hurts sharply, STOP. Honor your body's feedback and modify or seek professional guidance as needed.

Key Takeaways:

- **Celebrate Every Step:** Appreciate and take pride in even the smallest actions that move you towards your goals.
- **Find joy in the process:** When exercise feels enjoyable, it becomes a sustainable part of your life, bringing lasting change.
- **Be kind to yourself.** Some days will be easier than others. Show yourself compassion, adapt when needed, and keep going.

Conclusion

Embracing a Nourished Life – Your Transformation Awaits

Throughout this journey, we've illuminated the profound impact food choices have on our health and well-being. Let's recap the powerful principles that will guide you toward lasting, transformative change:

- **The Pitfalls of Processed Foods:** Packed with artificial ingredients, refined sugars, unhealthy fats, and lacking in essential nutrients, processed foods sabotage our health. Choosing whole, real foods empowers you to thrive.
- **The Power of Whole-Food Nutrition:** Nature's bounty abounds with fruits, vegetables, lean proteins, whole grains, and healthy fats – the foundations for optimal health. These foods nourish, protect against disease, and promote lasting energy and vitality.
- **Resetting with a Detox:** A properly designed detox plan can jump-start your journey, eliminating potential food sensitivities and reducing inflammation. It's a powerful tool for cultivating a deeper awareness of how food affects your body.
- **Nourishing Your Whole Self:** True nourishment extends beyond what's on your plate. Develop a mindful, positive relationship with food, one built on fueling your body and finding joy in healthy eating. Learn to listen to your hunger and fullness signals, fostering a sense

of empowerment around your choices.

- **Movement as Medicine:** Exercise is an invaluable partner to healthy eating. It boosts your metabolism, protects against chronic disease, enhances mood, strengthens your body, and maximizes your overall well-being. Find activities you enjoy – this is key to making it a lasting habit.

A Lifelong Journey

True transformation takes time and dedication. Remember:

- **Embrace the Process:** Sustainable change isn't about restrictive diets but about building a lifestyle that nourishes you for the long term.
- **Progress, Not Perfection:** There will be days when you slip up, and that's okay! Strive for progress, celebrate your victories, and extend compassion to yourself along the way.
- **Self-Love in Action:** Choosing whole foods, moving your body joyfully, and prioritizing your health are profound acts of self-care. Honor your body's incredible strength and resilience.

Call to Action

You already possess the potential to live a healthier, more vibrant life. Take the first step, however small:

- **Start with One Change:** Choose one area to focus on – swapping sugary drinks for water, adding more vegetables to your meals, or trying a new workout class.
- **Celebrate Your Wins:** Acknowledge every success, no matter how small. That boost of positive reinforcement fuels your motivation.

- **Gradual Wins the Race:** Focus on sustainable transformations instead of quick fixes that ultimately fail.

Inspiration and Ongoing Support

Remember the incredible benefits awaiting you on this journey: boosted energy levels, greater mental clarity, a stronger body, and reduced risk for chronic diseases. You deserve to feel your absolute best. Seek out support to fuel your path:

- **Trusted Resources:** Explore reliable websites and cookbooks dedicated to whole-food eating and healthy living.[You might want to provide specific examples]
- **Community Connection:** Join online communities or find a local group of like-minded individuals to share tips,recipes, and encouragement.

Your vibrant, healthy future starts today. Embrace the power of nourishment, celebrate your progress, and discover the joy of fueling your body and soul for a lifetime of well-being!

Appendix A: Recipes

Breakfast

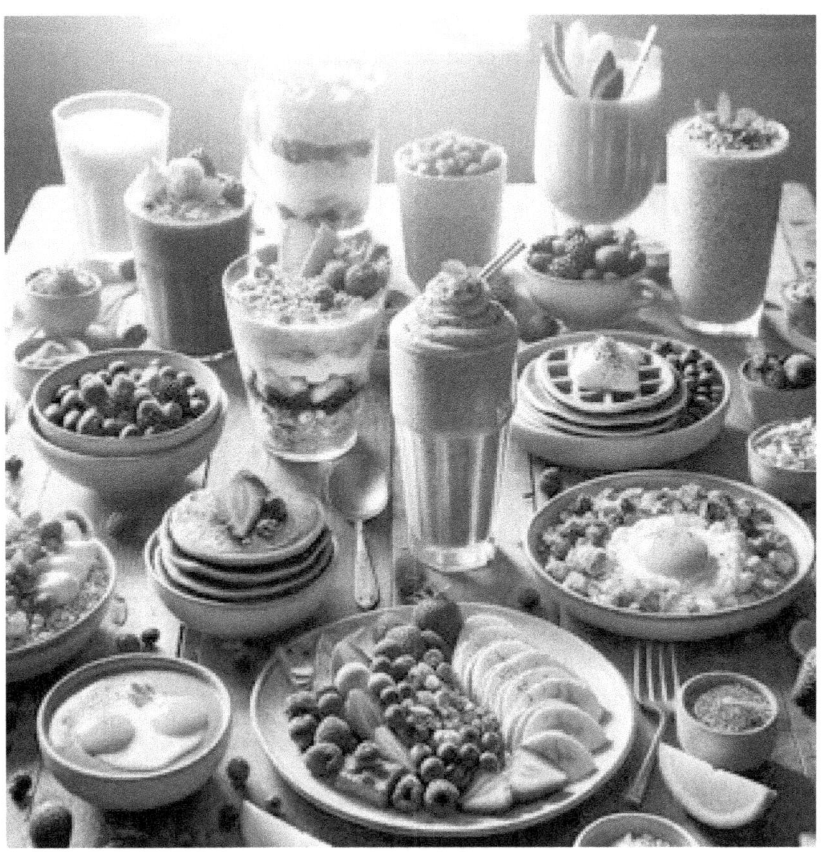

Overnight Oats Extravaganza

- Ingredients:
- 1/2 cup rolled oats
- 1/2 cup milk of choice (almond, oat, dairy, etc.)
- 1 tbsp chia seeds
- 1 tbsp maple syrup or honey (optional)
- 1/4 tsp vanilla extract
- Pinch of salt

- Toppings of your choice (see below)
- Instructions:

1. Combine all ingredients (except toppings) in a jar or container. Stir well.
2. Cover and refrigerate overnight (or at least 4 hours).
3. Top with your favorites: fresh berries, sliced banana, chopped nuts and seeds, nut butters, coconut flakes, etc. Get creative!

Berrylicious Smoothie

- Ingredients:
- 1 cup frozen mixed berries
- 1/2 cup spinach or kale
- 1/2 cup milk of choice
- 1 scoop protein powder (optional)
- 1 tbsp almond butter or peanut butter
- 1/4 tsp ground cinnamon
- Instructions:

1. Combine all ingredients in a blender and blend until smooth and creamy.
2. Adjust sweetness/thickness with additional milk or berries as needed.

Savory Egg Scramble

- Ingredients:
- 2 large eggs

- 1 tbsp olive oil
- 1/4 cup chopped onion
- 1/4 cup chopped bell pepper (any color)
- 1/2 cup chopped mushrooms
- Salt and pepper to taste
- Optional: grated cheese, fresh herbs for garnish
- Instructions:

1. Heat oil in a skillet. Add onions, bell peppers, mushrooms, and cook until softened.
2. Whisk eggs in a bowl, season with salt and pepper.
3. Pour eggs into the pan and scramble gently until cooked through. Top with cheese (if using) and herbs.

Sweet Potato Hash with Eggs

- Ingredients:
- 1 medium sweet potato, peeled and diced
- 1 tbsp olive oil
- 1/2 cup chopped onion
- 1/2 cup chopped red bell pepper
- 2 large eggs
- Salt, pepper, chili flakes to taste
- Optional: fresh cilantro for garnish
- Instructions:

1. Heat oil in a skillet. Cook diced sweet potato until tender, then add onions and bell peppers and cook until softened.
2. Create two wells in the pan, crack an egg into each. Season with salt, pepper, and chili flakes.

3. Cover pan and cook until eggs are set to your liking. Top with fresh cilantro.

Fluffy Yogurt Parfaits

- Ingredients:
- 1 cup plain Greek yogurt
- 1/2 cup granola (homemade or store-bought)
- 1 cup mixed berries
- Drizzle of honey or maple syrup
- Chopped nuts
- Instructions:

1. Layer yogurt, granola, and berries in glasses or jars.
2. Drizzle with honey or maple syrup and sprinkle on chopped nuts.

Whole Wheat Pancakes (or Waffles)

- Ingredients:
- 1 cup whole wheat flour
- 1 tbsp baking powder
- 1/2 tsp salt
- 1 egg
- 1 cup milk of choice
- 1 tbsp melted butter or oil
- Toppings: Fresh berries, maple syrup, nut butter
- Instructions:

1. Mix dry ingredients. Whisk together egg, milk, and oil. Add wet to

dry, mix until just combined (don't overmix).

2. Cook on a griddle or waffle iron. Top with your favorites.

Tofu Scramble

- Ingredients:
- 1 block extra-firm tofu, crumbled
- 1/4 cup chopped onion
- 1/4 cup chopped bell pepper
- 1/4 cup chopped mushrooms
- 1/4 tsp turmeric
- Salt, pepper, garlic powder to taste
- Optional: 2 tbsp nutritional yeast for cheesy flavor
- Instructions:

1. Heat a little oil in a skillet. Cook onions, peppers, and mushrooms until softened.
2. Add crumbled tofu, turmeric, and seasonings, cook until heated through, stirring occasionally.
3. Stir in nutritional yeast, if using.

Chia Seed Pudding

- Ingredients:
- 1/4 cup chia seeds
- 1 cup milk of choice
- 1 tbsp maple syrup or honey
- 1/2 tsp vanilla extract
- Toppings: Fresh fruit, nuts, seeds, coconut flakes
- Instructions:

1. Combine chia seeds, milk, sweetener, and vanilla. Stir well.
2. Cover and refrigerate overnight (or at least 4 hours). Top with desired toppings before serving.

Fruit & Yogurt Smoothie Bowl

- Ingredients:
- 1 cup frozen berries or fruit of choice
- 1/2 cup plain Greek yogurt
- 1/2 cup milk of choice
- 1 tbsp nut butter
- Toppings: granola, fresh fruit, chia seeds, honey
- Instructions:

1. Blend all ingredients (except toppings) until thick and creamy.
2. Pour into a bowl and top with your favorites for extra crunch and flavor.

Lunch

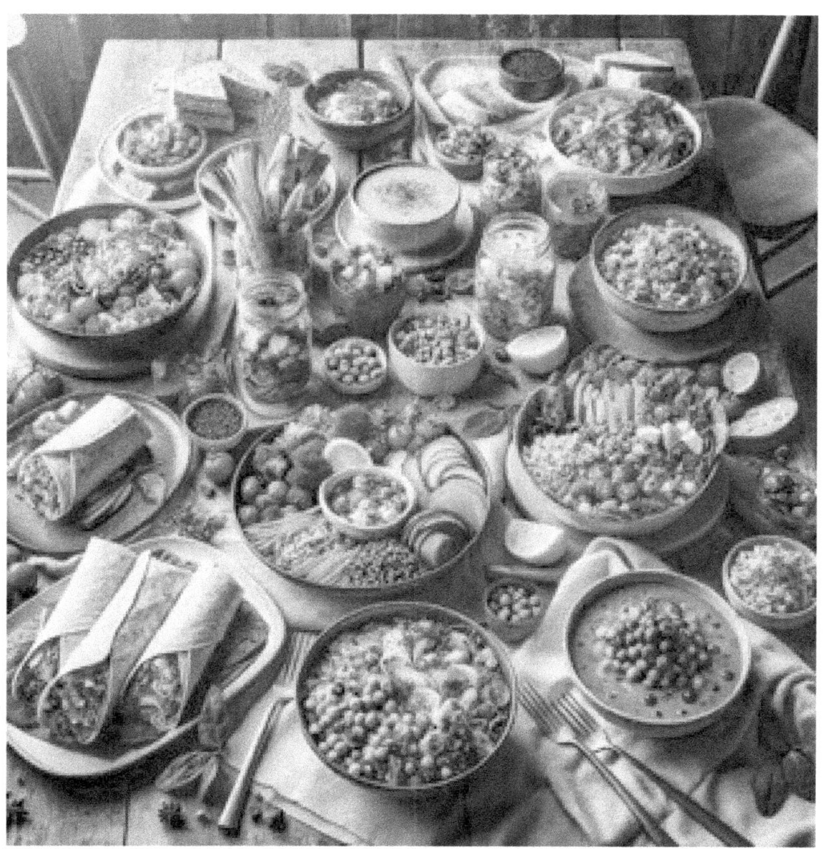

Rainbow Veggie Wraps

- Ingredients:
- Whole wheat or gluten-free tortillas
- Hummus
- Sliced cucumber
- Shredded carrots
- Bell pepper strips
- Avocado slices

- Handful of sprouts
- Optional: grilled chicken, baked tofu, or chickpeas
- Instructions:

1. Spread hummus on tortillas. Top with veggies and optional protein.
2. Roll tightly, slice in half, and enjoy!

Nourish Bowl Delight

- Ingredients:
- 1 cup cooked quinoa or brown rice
- 1/2 cup black beans or lentils (canned or pre-cooked)
- 1 cup roasted sweet potatoes or butternut squash
- Chopped tomato and cucumber
- Salsa
- Avocado slices
- Dollop of plain Greek yogurt (optional)
- Lime wedges, cumin, cilantro
- Instructions:

1. Assemble your bowl: base of grains, add beans/lentils, roasted veggies, tomato/cucumber, salsa, avocado, and yogurt.
2. Squeeze lime, sprinkle with cumin, and top with cilantro.

Supercharged Salad

- Ingredients:
- Mixed greens, spinach, or massaged kale
- Grilled salmon/chicken, chickpeas, or lentils
- Toasted sunflower/pumpkin seeds, chopped walnuts, crumbled

feta/goat cheese (optional)

- Dressing: Olive oil, balsamic vinegar, Dijon mustard, maple syrup/honey, salt, pepper
- Instructions:

1. Make the dressing: whisk all ingredients.
2. Assemble salad: base of greens, add protein, toppings, drizzle with dressing (store extra separately).

Mediterranean Chickpea Salad

- Ingredients:
- 1 can chickpeas, rinsed and drained
- Chopped cucumber, tomato, red onion
- Crumbled feta cheese (optional)
- Chopped fresh parsley or mint
- Dressing: Olive oil, lemon juice, salt, pepper
- Instructions:

1. Combine all ingredients in a bowl. Toss with dressing before serving.
2. Great as a sandwich filling, on top of greens, or with crackers!

Quinoa & Black Bean Salad

- Ingredients:
- 1 cup cooked quinoa
- 1 can black beans, rinsed and drained
- 1 cup chopped bell peppers

- 1/2 cup chopped cilantro
- Lime dressing: lime juice, olive oil, salt, pepper
- Instructions:

1. Combine all ingredients (except dressing) in a bowl. Whisk dressing and toss with salad.
2. Add corn kernels, avocado, or other favorite veggies for variation.

Lentil Soup

- Ingredients:
- 1 tbsp olive oil
- 1 onion, chopped
- 2 carrots, chopped
- 2 celery stalks, chopped
- 1 cup dried lentils, rinsed
- 4 cups vegetable broth
- 1 (14.5 oz) can diced tomatoes
- 1 tsp dried oregano
- Salt and pepper to taste
- Instructions:

1. Heat olive oil in a pot. Cook onions, carrots, celery until softened.
2. Add lentils, broth, tomatoes, oregano, salt, and pepper. Bring to a boil, reduce heat and simmer until lentils are tender (about 20-30 mins).

Black Bean Burgers (Vegetarian/Vegan)

- Ingredients:
- 1 can black beans, rinsed and drained
- 1/2 cup breadcrumbs
- 1/4 cup chopped onion
- 1/4 cup chopped cilantro
- 1 egg (or flax egg for vegan*)
- 1 tsp cumin
- Salt and pepper to taste
- Instructions:

1. Mash black beans. Mix in remaining ingredients. Form into patties.
2. Cook in a skillet with oil until browned, or bake at 400F. Serve on buns with your favorite toppings.*Flax egg: 1 tbsp flaxseed meal mixed with 3 tbsp water

Mediterranean Tuna Salad

- Ingredients:
- 1 can tuna, drained
- 1/2 cup chopped cucumber
- Chopped Kalamata olives
- Crumbled feta cheese
- Chopped fresh dill or parsley
- Dressing: Olive oil, red wine vinegar, salt, pepper
- Instructions:

1. Combine tuna, cucumber, olives, feta, herbs. Whisk dressing and toss with salad. Serve on greens,whole-grain bread, or with pita.

Chicken Caesar Salad Wraps

- Ingredients:
- Rotisserie chicken or leftover grilled chicken, shredded
- Romaine lettuce, chopped
- Grated Parmesan cheese
- Croutons
- Caesar dressing (bottled or homemade)
- Whole wheat or gluten-free tortillas
- Instructions:

1. Toss chicken, lettuce, parmesan, croutons, with dressing.
2. Spread on tortillas, roll up, and enjoy!

Roasted Veggie Pasta Salad

- Ingredients:
- Whole wheat or gluten-free pasta, cooked
- Roasted veggies of choice: zucchini, bell peppers, broccoli, etc.
- Cherry tomatoes, halved
- Fresh basil, chopped
- Dressing: Olive oil, balsamic vinegar, Dijon, honey/maple syrup, salt, pepper
- Instructions:

1. Toss cooked pasta with roasted veggies, tomatoes, and basil. Whisk dressing, toss with salad.

Mason Jar Salads

- Ingredients (ideas):

- Base: Quinoa, brown rice, lentils, greens
- Protein: Chicken, chickpeas, tofu
- Veggies: cucumbers, tomatoes, bell peppers, avocado... get creative!
- Crunch: Nuts, seeds, crumbled cheese
- Dressing (kept separate)
- Instructions:

1. Layer ingredients in mason jars, heaviest on the bottom, dressing on top. Keeps for days in fridge.
2. Dump into a bowl to eat, shake to distribute dressing.

Dinner

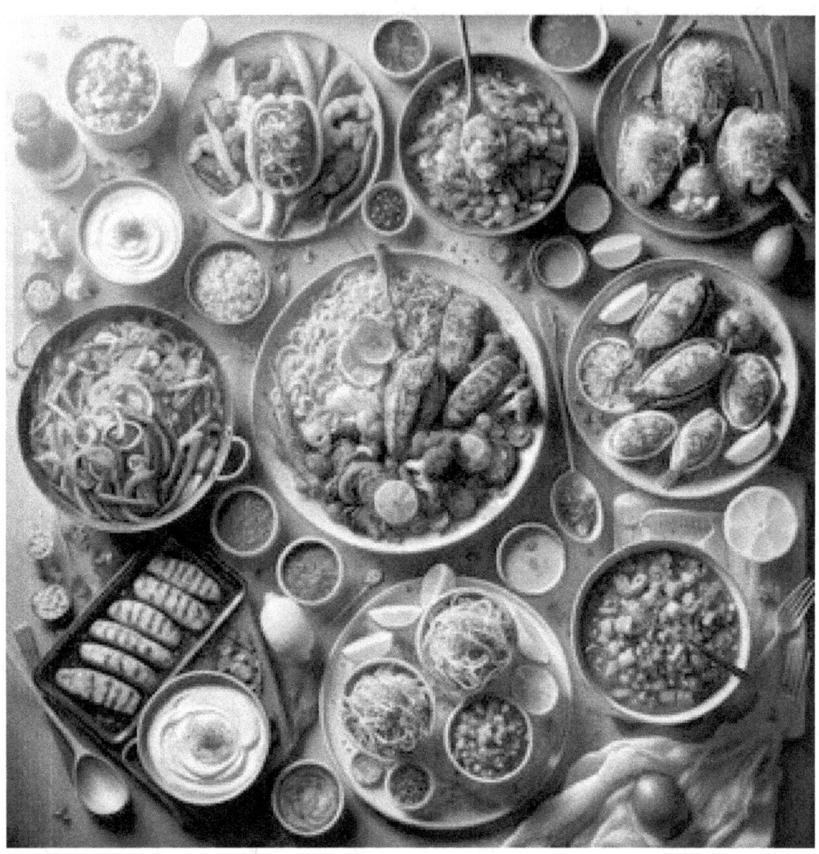

Chicken or Tofu Stir-Fry

- Ingredients:
- 1 lb diced chicken breast or extra-firm tofu
- Your favorite stir-fry veggies: broccoli, carrots, snow peas, bell peppers, etc.
- Sauce: soy sauce, rice vinegar, sesame oil, honey/maple syrup, ginger, garlic
- Rice or noodles for serving
- Instructions:

1. Cook chicken/tofu in a wok or skillet until browned. Set aside.
2. Stir-fry veggies until crisp-tender. Whisk sauce ingredients.
3. Return protein to pan with veggies, add sauce, and cook briefly until thickened. Serve over rice or noodles.

Vegetarian Stuffed Peppers

- Ingredients:
- 4 bell peppers, halved lengthwise
- Filling: cooked quinoa/rice, black beans, corn, chopped onion, tomato, spices (chili powder, cumin), shredded cheese
- Instructions:

1. Parboil peppers to soften slightly. Mix filling ingredients.
2. Stuff peppers with filling, top with cheese. Bake at 375F until peppers are tender and cheese is melted.

Shrimp Tacos with Avocado Salsa

- Ingredients:
- 1 lb shrimp, peeled and deveined
- Spices: chili powder, cumin, paprika, salt, pepper
- Corn or whole-wheat tortillas
- Salsa: diced avocado, tomato, onion, cilantro, lime juice
- Optional toppings: shredded cabbage, sour cream/plain yogurt
- Instructions:

1. Cook shrimp with spices in a skillet until pink.
2. Warm tortillas. Make avocado salsa. Assemble tacos with shrimp, salsa, and other toppings of choice.

One-Pan Roasted Chicken & Veggies

- Ingredients:
- Bone-in, skin-on chicken thighs or breasts
- 1 tbsp olive oil
- Salt, pepper, dried herbs (thyme, rosemary, Italian seasoning)
- Potatoes (any kind), cut into chunks
- Carrots, chopped
- Brussels sprouts, halved
- Instructions:

1. Preheat oven to 425°F. Toss chicken and veggies with oil, herbs, salt, and pepper.
2. Spread on a baking sheet. Roast for 30-40 minutes, or until chicken is cooked through and veggies are tender.

Sheet Pan Salmon with Lemon & Dill

- Ingredients:
- 1 lb salmon fillet
- 1 tbsp olive oil
- Lemon wedges
- Salt, pepper, dried dill
- Asparagus spears or broccoli florets
- Sliced red onion
- Instructions:

1. Preheat oven to 400°F. Place salmon on a baking sheet lined with parchment paper.
2. Toss veggies with oil, salt, pepper, spread on the sheet. Top salmon with lemon wedges, dill, salt, pepper.

3. Roast 12–15 minutes, or until salmon is cooked through and veggies tender.

Shrimp Scampi with Whole Wheat Pasta

- Ingredients:
- 1 lb shrimp, peeled and deveined
- 1/2 cup whole wheat pasta
- 2 tbsp olive oil
- 4 cloves garlic, minced
- 1/4 cup white wine or broth
- Juice of 1 lemon
- Small handful fresh spinach
- Crushed red pepper flakes, salt, pepper
- Instructions:

1. Cook pasta. Heat oil in a skillet, add garlic, cook until fragrant. Add shrimp, season, cook until pink.
2. Add wine/broth, lemon juice, red pepper flakes, spinach. Simmer briefly.
3. Toss cooked pasta with shrimp and sauce.

Vegetarian Chili

- Ingredients:
- 1 tbsp olive oil
- 1 onion, chopped
- 2 bell peppers, chopped
- 2 cloves garlic, minced
- 1 (15oz) can black beans, rinsed
- 1 (15oz) can kidney beans, rinsed

- 1 (14.5oz) can diced tomatoes
- 2 cups vegetable broth
- Spices: chili powder, cumin, paprika, salt, pepper
- Instructions:

1. Heat oil in a pot. Cook onion and peppers until softened. Add garlic and cook briefly.
2. Add beans, tomatoes, broth, spices. Simmer for 30 minutes to allow flavors to blend.

Turkey Meatballs with Marinara

- Ingredients:
- 1 lb ground turkey
- 1/2 cup breadcrumbs
- 1/4 cup grated Parmesan cheese
- 1 egg
- Dried oregano, basil, salt, pepper
- Your favorite jarred marinara sauce
- Whole wheat pasta or zucchini noodles
- Instructions:

1. Combine meatball ingredients. Form into meatballs. Brown in a skillet with a bit of oil, or bake at 400F.
2. Cook pasta (or spiralize zucchini). Heat marinara and add meatballs. Simmer briefly. Serve over pasta/zoodles.

Biryani-Inspired Lentil Bowls

- Ingredients:
- 1 cup cooked lentils

- Cooked rice or quinoa
- Sautéed veggies: onions, bell peppers, mushrooms, spinach
- Spices: Curry powder, turmeric, cumin, salt, pepper
- Plain yogurt for dolloping
- Diced cucumber and tomato
- Chopped cilantro
- Instructions:

1. Sauté veggies with spices. Build your bowl: base of rice/quinoa, add lentils, spiced veggies, top with yogurt, cucumber/tomato, cilantro.

Baked Tofu with Peanut Sauce

- Ingredients:
- 1 block extra-firm tofu, pressed, cut into cubes
- Sauce: Peanut butter, soy sauce, rice vinegar, sesame oil, maple syrup/honey, ginger, sriracha (optional)
- Veggies of choice for stir-fry: broccoli, carrots, bell peppers...
- Instructions:

1. Toss tofu in a mix of cornstarch, salt, pepper. Bake at 400F until crispy.
2. Whisk sauce ingredients. Stir fry veggies. Serve cooked rice/quinoa, topped with tofu, veggies, and sauce.

Snacks

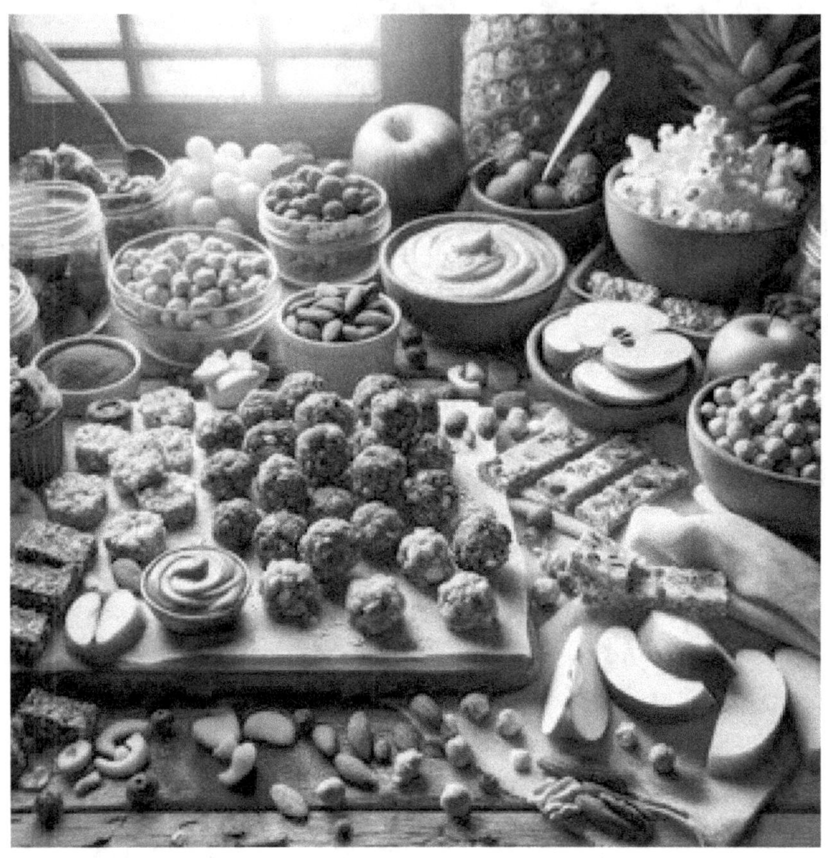

Energy Bites

- Ingredients:
- 1 cup rolled oats
- 1/2 cup nut butter
- 1/4 cup honey or maple syrup
- 1/4 cup flaxseeds or chia seeds
- 1/2 cup mix-ins: chopped nuts, dried fruit, coconut flakes, etc.
- Instructions:

1. Combine all ingredients. Roll into balls, chill in the fridge.

Apple Slices with Almond Butter & Cinnamon

- Ingredients:
- 1 apple, sliced
- Almond butter
- Sprinkle of cinnamon

Roasted Chickpeas

- Ingredients:
- Can of chickpeas, rinsed, patted dry
- Olive oil, salt, pepper, spices of choice (paprika, cumin, garlic powder, etc.)
- Instructions:

1. Toss chickpeas with oil and spices. Roast at 400F until crispy (about 20 mins)

Fruit & Nut Yogurt Bark

- Ingredients:
- Plain Greek yogurt
- Berries or chopped fruit
- Chopped nuts or seeds
- Drizzle of honey or maple syrup (optional)
- Instructions:

1. Spread yogurt on a parchment-lined baking sheet. Top with fruit, nuts/seeds, a drizzle of honey (if desired).

2. Freeze until solid. Break into pieces and enjoy!

Veggies & Hummus

- Ingredients:
- Sliced carrots, celery sticks, bell pepper strips, cucumber rounds, snap peas
- Hummus (store-bought or homemade)

Hard-Boiled Eggs

- Ingredients:
- Hard-boiled eggs, peeled and sliced
- Sprinkle of Everything But the Bagel seasoning (or your favorite spice mix)

Greek Yogurt with Granola and Fruit

- Ingredients:
- Plain Greek yogurt
- Granola
- Fresh or frozen berries

Trail Mix

- Ingredients:
- Mixed nuts
- Dried fruits (no added sugar)
- Seeds (pumpkin, sunflower)
- Unsweetened coconut flakes (optional)
- Dark chocolate chips (optional, small amount)

- Instructions:
- Combine your favorite ingredients in a jar or baggie, portion out for on-the-go snacks.

Popcorn

- Ingredients:
- Popcorn kernels, air-popped
- Small drizzle of melted butter or olive oil (optional)
- Toppings: Nutritional yeast, sprinkle of Parmesan, salt, herbs... experiment!

Rice Cakes with Toppings

- Ingredients:
- Brown rice cakes
- Topping Ideas: Nut butter & sliced banana, avocado & salt, hummus & sliced veggies, cream cheese & cucumber

Recipes Designed with Adaptability in Mind

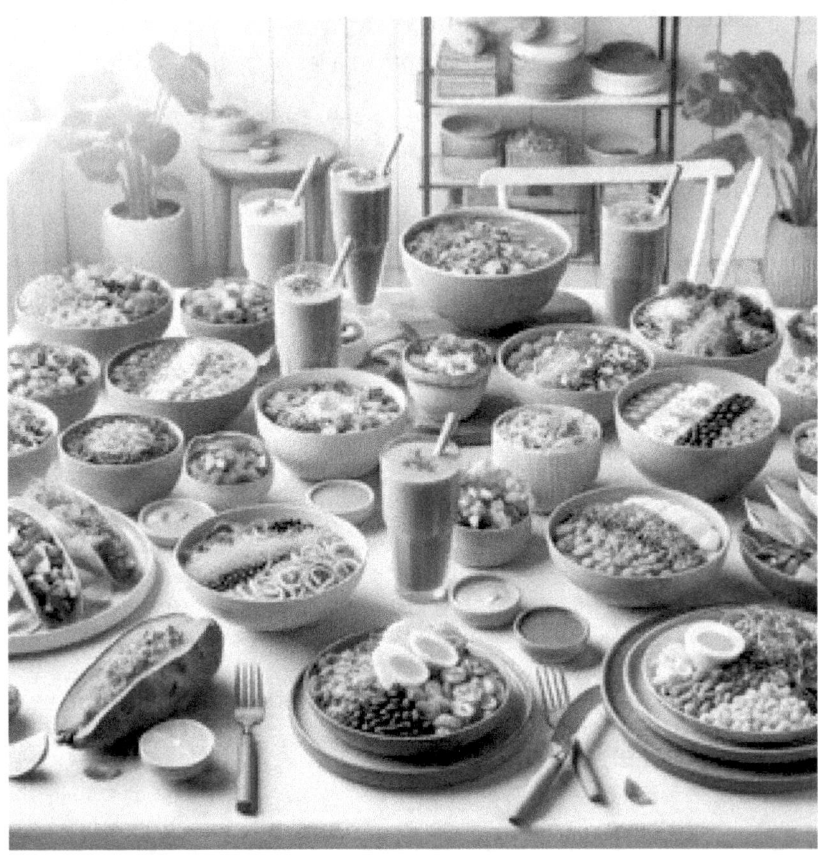

Customizable Grain Bowls

- **Base:**
- Cooked grain of choice: Quinoa, brown rice, farro, or use gluten-free options if needed.
- **Protein:**
- Grilled/baked chicken or tofu
- Lentils or beans (seasoned however you like)
- Poached or baked fish

- **Veggies:**
- Mix and match! Roasted, raw, sautéed... the options are limitless! Choose your favorites or what's in season.
- **Sauce/Dressing:**
- Tahini-lemon
- Peanut sauce
- Balsamic vinaigrette
- Yogurt-based herb sauce
- **Instructions:** Assemble bowls with a base of grain, add protein, veggies, and drizzle with your chosen sauce.

Veggie-Packed Soup

- **Base:**
- Olive oil, onion, celery, carrots (the classic aromatic trio)
- Vegetable or chicken broth
- Diced tomatoes (canned or fresh)
- Spices: Adjust to taste – Italian herbs, cumin, chili powder, etc.
- **Add-Ins:**
- Lentils, beans, or chickpeas
- Potatoes, sweet potatoes, or winter squash
- Chopped kale, spinach, or other greens
- **Instructions:**

1. Sauté aromatics. Add broth, tomatoes, spices.
2. Simmer with lentils/beans/potatoes until tender.
3. Stir in greens near the end. Season to taste and enjoy!

Stuffed Sweet Potatoes

- **Base:** Roasted sweet potatoes

- **Filling Options:**
- Black beans, corn, salsa, avocado, cheese (optional) – Mexican-inspired
- Cooked chickpeas, spinach, feta, drizzle of Greek yogurt – Mediterranean vibes
- Ground chicken/turkey cooked with taco seasoning
- **Instructions:**

1. Bake sweet potatoes until tender.
2. Mash flesh slightly, scoop in your chosen filling, top with any desired extras.

Customizable Pasta

- **Pasta:** Choose whole-wheat, gluten-free (lentil, chickpea, etc.), or zucchini noodles for a veggie-forward option.
- **Sauce:**
- Simple marinara (can be homemade or jarred)
- Pesto (store-bought or try making your own)
- Olive oil, garlic, lemon juice, Parmesan, and chopped greens
- **Protein/Veggies:**
- Grilled chicken or shrimp
- Sautéed mushrooms, spinach, broccoli – get creative!
- White beans or chickpeas for vegetarian-friendly boost
- **Instructions:** Cook pasta, toss with your chosen sauce and additions.

Egg-Based Frittata

- **Base:**
- Eggs whisked with a splash of milk or cream (dairy-free options work too)

- Salt, pepper, and any herbs you like
- **Fillings:** Endless possibilities!
- Sautéed onions, mushrooms, spinach
- Crumbled feta cheese, chopped tomatoes
- Cooked sausage or bacon (omit for vegetarian)
- Leftover roasted vegetables
- **Instructions:**

1. Sauté any fillings. Pour egg mixture into an oven-safe skillet.
2. Top with fillings. Bake at 350F until set.

Tacos or Lettuce Wraps

- **Tortillas/Lettuce:** Corn or whole-wheat tortillas, or large lettuce leaves for lower-carb option
- **Filling:**
- Ground turkey/chicken cooked with your favorite spice mix
- Beans or lentils with Mexican-inspired seasonings
- Baked or grilled fish (think blackened or Cajun-style)
- Crispy tofu crumbles
- **Toppings:**
- Avocado or guacamole
- Salsa (mild to spicy)
- Shredded cheese, sour cream, or plain yogurt
- Shredded cabbage or lettuce
- **Instructions:** Assemble with your chosen fillings and toppings.

Smoothies

- **Base:** Milk of choice, plain yogurt (Greek for extra protein)
- **Flavor Boosters:**

- Frozen fruit (berries, banana, mango, etc.)
- Scoop of protein powder
- Handful of spinach or kale
- Nut butters, chia seeds, flaxseeds
- **Instructions:** Blend and enjoy!

Appendix B:Food Swaps

Goodbye Processed, Hello Nourishing!

Processed foods are often laden with unhealthy fats, refined sugars, sodium, and artificial ingredients. Here's how to break free and replace those common culprits with delicious and nourishing alternatives:

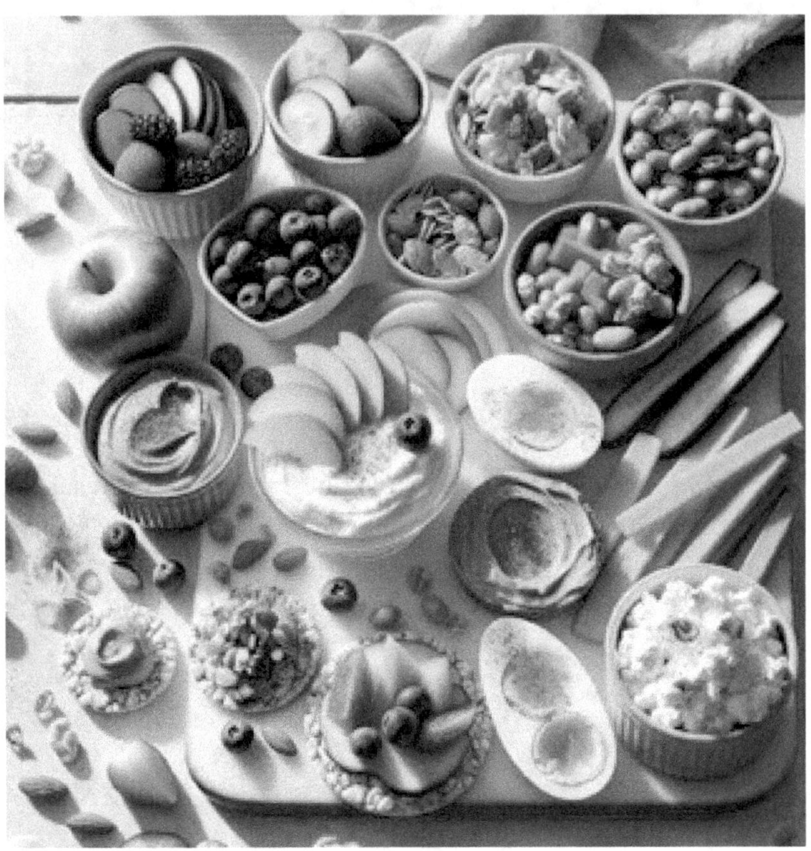

Chips & Crackers

- **Instead of:** Store-bought chips and crackers, often high in sodium and unhealthy fats.
- **Try:**
- Homemade Kale Chips: Toss kale with olive oil, salt, and spices. Bake until crispy.
- Roasted Chickpeas: Toss chickpeas with olive oil, salt, and spices. Roast until crunchy.

- Sliced Veggies: Cucumbers, bell peppers, carrots – great for dipping into hummus or guacamole.
- Air-Popped Popcorn: Lightly drizzle with olive oil or melted butter, and sprinkle with nutritional yeast or Parmesan cheese.
- Rice Cakes: Choose whole-grain versions and top with nut butter, avocado, or sliced veggies.

Dressings & Sauces

- **Instead of:** Bottled salad dressings, marinades, and sauces, often loaded with sugar, unhealthy oils, and preservatives.
- **Try:**
- Simple Vinaigrette: Whisk together olive oil, balsamic vinegar, Dijon mustard, a touch of honey, salt, and pepper.
- Tahini Dressing: Blend tahini, lemon juice, garlic, water, salt, and pepper.
- Yogurt-Based Dressings: Mix plain Greek yogurt with herbs, lemon juice, and spices.
- Blended Pesto: Fresh basil, pine nuts, Parmesan cheese, garlic, olive oil – classic and versatile.
- Homemade Marinara: Sautéed onions, garlic, canned tomatoes, herbs – healthier than most jarred versions.

Satisfying Cravings with Whole Foods

- **Sweet Cravings:**
- Fruit Salad: Mix your favorites for a natural burst of sweetness.
- Fruit with Plain Yogurt: Add a drizzle of honey and a sprinkle of granola for a satisfying treat.
- Dark Chocolate Covered Fruit: Dip strawberries, banana slices, or dried fruit for a decadent yet healthier indulgence.

- Energy Bites: Made with oats, nut butter, dried fruit, and seeds for a naturally sweet pick-me-up.
- Nice Cream: Frozen bananas blended into a creamy, healthier "ice cream" base.
- **Savory & Salty Cravings:**
- Nuts and Seeds: Almonds, cashews, walnuts, pistachios, pumpkin seeds, sunflower seeds.
- Hard-Boiled Eggs: A sprinkle of Everything But the Bagel seasoning adds savory flavor.
- Avocado Toast: Smashed avocado on whole-grain toast, topped with salt, pepper, and red pepper flakes.
- Olives or Pickles: Provide a satisfying salty and tangy bite.
- Soup: A hearty broth-based vegetable soup can tame savory cravings healthily.

Healthy Snack Inspiration

1. Apple slices with almond butter
2. Plain Greek yogurt with berries and granola
3. Hummus with veggie sticks (carrots, bell peppers, cucumbers)
4. Roasted edamame with a sprinkle of salt
5. Cottage cheese with sliced tomato and cucumber
6. Small handful of trail mix (nuts, seeds, dried fruit)
7. Rice cake with avocado and a sprinkle of red pepper flakes
8. Tuna salad on whole-grain crackers
9. Sliced hard-boiled egg with a sprinkle of paprika
10. A piece of fruit and a cheese stick

Key Points:

- **Prep in Advance:** Having healthy snacks ready eliminates resorting to processed options.

- **Experiment:** Discover flavor combinations you enjoy!
- **Mindful Eating:** Pay attention to your body's cues for hunger and satisfaction.

Appendix C: Glossary of Nutritional Terms

Understanding the Building Blocks

Macronutrients (Macros): The three main nutrients your body needs in large quantities for energy and vital functions.

- Carbohydrates: The primary fuel source. Types include sugars, starches (grains, potatoes), and fiber.
- Protein: Building blocks for muscles, tissues, and enzymes. Found in meat, poultry, fish, beans, lentils, tofu,eggs, nuts, and seeds.
- Fats: Provide energy, insulate the body, and aid nutrient absorption. Sources include avocados, nuts, seeds,olive oil, and fatty fish.

Micronutrients: Vitamins and minerals, needed in smaller amounts but essential for countless bodily processes.Found abundantly in fruits, vegetables, whole grains, and animal-based foods.

Health-Protective Compounds

Antioxidants: Protect cells from damage caused by free radicals (unstable molecules). Found in colorful fruits,vegetables, tea, and dark chocolate. Examples include vitamin C, vitamin E, and beta-carotene.

- **Phytonutrients:** Plant-based compounds with potential health benefits. Not considered essential nutrients but may play a role in disease prevention. Found in brightly colored fruits, vegetables, whole grains, and legumes. Examples include lycopene (tomatoes) and flavonoids (berries).
- **Fiber:** The indigestible part of plant foods. Key for digestive health, blood sugar control, and feeling satisfied.There are two types:
- Soluble Fiber: Dissolves in water, found in oats, beans, apples, citrus fruits
- Insoluble Fiber: Doesn't dissolve, promotes healthy bowel movements. Found in whole grains, nuts,vegetables.

Deciphering Food Labels

- **Calories:** A unit of energy. Food provides calories, your body burns them for fuel.
- **Serving Size:** The recommended portion of a food listed on the Nutrition Facts label.
- **% Daily Value (%DV):** Indicates how much of a nutrient a serving provides based on a 2,000 calorie diet. Helps gauge if a food is high or low in a specific nutrient.
- **Ingredients:** Listed in descending order by weight. Helps identify less obvious sources of sugar, unhealthy fats, and additives.

Additional Helpful Terms

- **Whole Foods:** Foods in their natural state or minimally processed. Examples include fruits, vegetables, whole grains, legumes, nuts, and seeds.
- **Processed Foods:** Foods that have undergone alterations from their natural state. Can range from minimally processed (washed

and bagged spinach) to ultra-processed (packaged snacks, sugary drinks).

- **Organic:** Food grown and produced according to specific standards, including minimizing synthetic pesticides and fertilizers.
- **Gluten-Free:** Excluding the protein gluten, found in wheat, rye, and barley. Important for those with Celiac disease or gluten sensitivity.
- **Added Sugars:** Sugars added during processing, not naturally occurring (like in fruit). Look for these on the ingredients list (corn syrup, dextrose, etc.).
- **Trans Fats:** Harmful fats made through processing. Should be avoided as much as possible. Found in some processed baked goods, fried foods, and margarines.

Key Takeaways

- **Knowledge is Power:** Understanding these terms empowers you to make informed dietary choices.
- **Focus on Whole Foods:** Prioritize whole foods, which naturally pack in essential nutrients and protective compounds.
- **Read Food Labels:** They can be a helpful tool, especially when choosing packaged goods.

Appendix D: Recommended Resources

Reliable Websites for Nutrition Information:

Government Agencies:

- United States Department of Agriculture (USDA): (https://www.myplate.gov/): Provides evidence-based guidelines, recipes, and information about MyPlate (visual representation of a healthy meal).
- The Academy of Nutrition and Dietetics (AND): (https://www.eatright.org/): The largest organization of food and nutrition professionals. Find a registered dietitian in your area, credible articles, and practical tips.
- Centers for Disease Control and Prevention (CDC): (https://www.cdc.gov/healthyweight/index.html):Focuses on healthy weight management, disease prevention, and reliable health information.

Reputable Institutions:

- The Mayo Clinic: (https://www.mayoclinic.org/healthy-lifestyle): Offers reliable information on diet,exercise, and conditions related to nutrition.
- The Cleveland Clinic: (https://my.clevelandclinic.org/health/disea

ses): Trusted resource for articles on specific health conditions and how nutrition plays a role.

- Harvard T.H. Chan School of Public Health: (https://www.hsph .harvard.edu/nutritionsource/): Provides cutting-edge research, debunks nutrition myths, and offers practical healthy eating advice.

Highly Recommended Books:

- **"How Not to Die" by Dr. Michael Greger:** Explores the power of whole-food, plant-based eating for preventing and reversing chronic diseases, backed by scientific research.
- **"Intuitive Eating" by Evelyn Tribole and Elyse Resch:** A non-diet approach, promoting a healthy relationship with food, body image, and mindful eating.
- **"Food Rules" by Michael Pollan:** Simple, practical guidelines for making healthier food choices. Focus on whole foods and cooking at home.
- **"The Blue Zones Kitchen" by Dan Buettner:** Explore dietary patterns of regions with exceptional longevity, offering recipes and inspiration for healthy, plant-focused eating.
- **"In Defense of Food" by Michael Pollan:** Examines the negative impact of the Western diet and processed foods, advocating for a return to whole foods.

Finding Individualized Support:

- **Registered Dietitian Nutritionists (RDNs) / Registered Dietitians (RDs):** Credentialed professionals with expertise in translating nutrition science into individualized plans. Find one through the Academy of Nutrition and Dietetics (https://www.eatright.org/): Ideal for those with specific health concerns, food allergies, or wanting in-depth guidance.

- **Certified Nutrition Specialists (CNS):** Professionals with advanced degrees in nutrition. Focus on whole-food,personalized plans. May have varying expertise, so inquire about their areas of focus.
- **Health Coaches:** Can support in setting goals, habit change, and offer accountability. Backgrounds vary, so ensure they have a solid grounding in nutrition principles.

Additional Considerations

- **Community Programs:** Check local hospitals, fitness centers, or government agencies for cooking classes,nutrition workshops, or support groups.
- **Online Communities and Forums:** Connect with like-minded individuals for support, recipe sharing, and motivation.
- **Reputable Food Blogs:** Many run by RDNs or focused on healthy eating. Examples include: Ambitious Kitchen,Cookie and Kate, Eating Bird Food.

Important Reminder: Always consider the source of information and prioritize sources based on scientific evidence and reputable credentials.

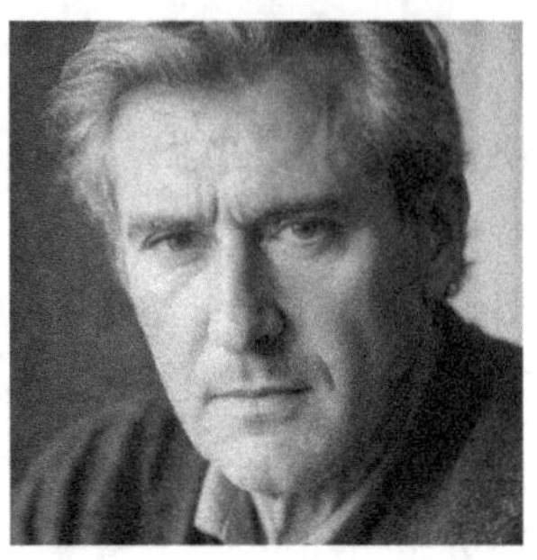

About the Author

Mike Barrel, the imaginative mind behind a series of bestselling cooking books, has carved a niche in the culinary literary world. Born into a family with a deep-rooted passion for food, Mike's journey into gastronomy began at an early age. Growing up amidst the aromas of his grandmother's kitchen, he developed an insatiable curiosity for diverse cuisines and cooking techniques. Mike's wanderlust led him to explore culinary traditions across the globe, from the bustling markets of Marrakech to the intimate kitchens of Tokyo. His adventurous spirit and dedication to capturing the essence of each culinary experience are evident in his engaging narratives.